Rachel Carr was born in Hankow,
China, and has spent the greater part of
her life in the Orient. A serious follower
of yoga, she has written extensively on
this subject, adopting its practical aspects
to the needs of adults and children.

Inspired to write *ARTHRITIS Relief
Beyond Drugs* after her own successful
battle with osteo-arthritis, the author is
now free from pain and has achieved a
flexibility and strength anyone might
envy.

Although there is no miracle cure for
arthritis, those afflicted can do much to
help themselves, and in this book, Rachel
Carr shares with sufferers the simple and
natural techniques she used in her victory
over the disease.

ARTHRITIS
Relief Beyond Drugs

Rachel Carr

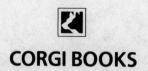

CORGI BOOKS

ARTHRITIS Relief Beyond Drugs

A CORGI BOOK 0 552 99033 7

First publication in Great Britain

PRINTING HISTORY
Corgi edition published 1983

Portions of this work originally appeared in *Woman's Day*.

Grateful acknowledgment is made for permission to reprint:

The three drawings of joints on page 28 by Neil O. Hardy, from *Reader's Digest Family Health Guide and Medical Encyclopedia*, page 488. Copyright © 1970 by The Reader's Digest Association, Inc.

Photographs on pages 57 and 60 by Nancy Brown, courtesy of *Woman's Day*.

Illustrations on pages 35, 36, 37 from *Human Anatomy and Physiology*, 6th ed., by B.G. King and M.J. Showers. Published by W.B. Saunders Co., Philadelphia, 1969.

This book is set in 11/12 Mallard

Corgi Books are published by
Transworld Publishers Ltd.,
Century House, 61–63 Uxbridge Road,
Ealing, London W5 5SA

Made and printed in Great Britain by the
Guernsey Press Co. Ltd., Guernsey, Channel Islands.

Introduction

As a rheumatologist I frequently have to break the news to a patient that he or she is suffering from arthritis. Fortunately, most arthritic patients do not become seriously disabled and a good many rheumatic conditions improve with time. There are, however, no miracle cures and most patients, even with mild arthritis, need help in coming to terms with their condition and need to know what they can do to help themselves. Anyone who finds himself in this situation should be helped by Rachel Carr's book. Here she describes her own battle against osteo-arthritis and the great benefit she and others have gained from her exercise programme. She rightly emphasises the importance of mental attitudes to physical suffering and includes descriptions of relaxation techniques, as well as exercises to strengthen and mobilise affected joints. There is something here for all arthritic sufferers, including a useful section for those with that very common complaint, low back pain. A number of passive exercises are also described, which can be used by a friend or relative to help those with severe crippling arthritis.

This book should prove valuable, both for the detailed exercises outlined here and the encouragement of Rachel Carr's own victory over disability.

Dr. Anthea Howell M.R.C.P.
Rheumatologist

CONTENTS

ACKNOWLEDGMENTS

I owe special thanks to Dr. H. Vann Austin, specialist in rheumatology, for his critical reading of this manuscript in its early stages, and for his invaluable assistance.

My gratitude is also extended to Dr. Jane E. Oltman, psychiatrist, for her comments on mind-control exercises for the arthritis sufferer.

I would like to express my appreciation to Jeanne Flagg of Harper & Row for her interest in the manuscript and her creative editing.

The people who appear in these pages are all personal friends who have been generous with their time in posing for the different exercises. While not all of them are afflicted with arthritis, many have found these physical and mental disciplines extremely helpful in easing the normal aches and pains of the body, as well as in releasing tension.

This book would not have been possible without the assistance of my husband, Edward Kimball, who spent endless hours taking the photographs.

FOREWORD

As a psychiatrist I have often wished for a book that my patients suffering from the discomfort and anxiety of joint pain could use on their own. Low back pain is the most common joint problem referred to psychiatrists. Many of us find that the condition can be relieved not only through psychotherapy and relaxation, but by regular exercises as well. Some physicians prescribe exercises for chronic ills without giving explicit instructions. Patients are frequently reluctant to bother their medical doctors, yet feel free to discuss their needs for more instructions with their psychiatrists. Rachel Carr's simple approach to natural therapy through physical and mental exercises provides this guidance—and more.

The chapter on passive exercises is especially valuable for the willing relative or friend who needs clear and concise instructions to help the sufferer. Patients at rehabilitation centers will greatly benefit from the supplementary therapy described here that they can do on their own.

This important handbook is the answer to the most common advice given today by physicians to their arthritis patients: 'Learn to live with it.' But how? Many of the answers can be found in the pages of this book.

JANE E. OLTMAN, M.D.

PREFACE

Treatment of the arthritis patient involves many aspects of care. Since the amount of time spent with the physician is necessarily limited, even with frequent office visits, it is important that patients understand the disease process and learn how to carry out any home self-care measures that might lead to improvement of their condition.

When a patient is first seen by a rheumatologist, a diagnosis is made and a program of therapy is worked out. Frequently, two basic questions must be addressed immediately: In which joints can motion be improved, and in what areas should stretching and muscle toning be instituted to preserve joint movement? Thus the patient is involved from the start in a self-help program that comes under the general heading of physical therapy. The benefits of such self-help can be considerable, not the least of which is the patient's feeling—and rightly so—that 'I can do something to help myself.'

Rachel Carr's book can be of great value to arthritis patients who are or can be motivated to help themselves. Here is a variety of specific programs for improving and preserving joint motion and for toning joint area muscles. Her emphasis on attitude training and adjustment, an aspect of treatment often overlooked, is commendable. To people with chronic pain from arthritis, attitude makes a significant difference in the level of discomfort. Some patients have severe arthritis but little pain, others mild arthritis but high levels of pain. This may seem to be a contradiction, but it is not surprising once we remember that pain is perceived in the brain cortex. In other words, the brain is involved in 'feeling pain'; therefore, the perception of pain can be modified.

Unquestionably, attitude adjustment can be the most important part of the treatment program for patients with chronic arthritis pain.

H. VANN AUSTIN, M.D.

A LETTER TO ARTHRITIS SUFFERERS

If you are among the millions of people suffering from arthritis, you can do a great deal to help yourself. Since there are well over a hundred different conditions that carry the label 'arthritis,' and many stages of each, it is important to get a competent medical diagnosis of the type you have.

While drug therapy is essential for the more serious cases of arthritis, drugs alone are not enough. Equally essential are physical and mental disciplines that you can do for yourself. By these means, the emotional effects of chronic pain and mental depression can be greatly reduced. Your body and mind have tremendous recuperative powers and they will respond to the therapeutic exercises outlined here.

While this book offers no miracle cure, it will make you aware of how you can help yourself. With advice from your doctor as to the types of exercises you should do, chart them in a daily program, preferably fifteen minutes twice a day to keep your joints mobile. These exercises are not calisthenics and must be done slowly so you can feel each stretch of a muscle and loosening of a joint. When you learn to breathe deeply and rhythmically, you will become much more relaxed. The effort will pay off if you are serious about exercising daily. You will see results within a few weeks: the pain in your joints will lessen; you will be able to bend lower, reach higher, stretch further. From this increased mobility you will gain a sense of exhilaration. As your stamina and flexibility improve, you will be able to incorporate wider ranges of movement. Even if you have the crippling type of arthritis, there are many helpful passive exercises that someone can do with you.

The Arthritis Foundation reminds us that while arthritis is a chronic condition, it can be treated and the range of movement can be increased. Disabilities can be prevented before they occur, and often effectively reduced if they have occurred already. When painful joints are kept for long periods in what feels like a comfortable position, they may become frozen and muscles around the joints may weaken from inactivity. The way to keep joints mobile is to move them. 'No case is hopeless,' says the Arthritis Foundation. 'Something can be done for every patient. The best possible solution to relieve pain and increase flexibility in the joints is a balanced proportion of rest and exercise. Too much inactivity can cause stiffening of the joints and limit the range of movement. Many arthritics become needlessly disabled.'

I have been inspired to write this book as a result of my personal battle with osteoarthritis. Dramatic things can sometimes be made to happen through the desire to help ourselves. The mind is a powerful instrument. It can make or break us. When it is tranquil it can push our anxieties away. Set toward a goal, it can overcome enormous obstacles.

RACHEL CARR

ARTHRITIS
Relief Beyond Drugs

1 MY VICTORY OVER ARTHRITIS

My battle with arthritis began when I was in my early twenties. I was living in China, where I was born and grew up. The first symptom was pressure on the nerves along my spinal cord. The only way I could sit with a minimum of discomfort was at the edge of a hard seat. X-rays showed an injury of the two lower vertebrae, possibly from a childhood accident. I learned that I had osteoarthritis, the most common type, and that no known treatment would cure the condition. The large doses of aspirin I took to cope with the pain eventually caused internal bleeding.

'If it is any consolation to you,' the doctor told me, 'you are indeed fortunate you don't have rheumatoid arthritis. That's the crippling kind.'

When I left China for Tokyo early in 1950 I consulted an orthopedist. X-rays showed further deterioration of the spine. He prescribed traction. Forty pounds of weight pulled on my back while I slept on a hard surface. The nights were long and sleepless, with little relief. After four agonizing years, the traction was abandoned for cortisone injections. This treatment was abruptly stopped when my intolerance to the drug was discovered. The pain spread with full force, paralyzing me at times. I took to bed, but total inactivity brought about a host of new problems. Depression topped them all. Lack of exercise caused my joints to become frozen. My fingers and ankles grew stiff and painful. The

17

years passed with no relief from physical and mental suffering.

In the 1960s when I made my new home in New York City, I saw an arthritis specialist. He looked at the last X-rays I had had taken in Tokyo and told me that the calcification in my spine had increased. When he learned of my intolerance to drugs, he tried X-ray treatment. The reaction was violent: it caused severe vomiting, and the muscle relaxants he prescribed made me continually depressed.

'There is nothing further I can do to help you,' the doctor said. 'Learn to live with your disability.'

It was my last visit. My spirits sank to the lowest possible depth. I began to question whether the pain was real or not. Was I a hypochondriac? Was I imagining these shooting pains in my body? Why was I continually depressed? My weight dropped from 106 to 95 pounds, and preoccupation with my failing condition became obsessive. A friend who watched this slow degeneration suggested I meet Yogi Vithaldas, a well-traveled man who has taught hundreds of people natural ways of healing the body and using the power of the mind. Among the more famous individuals he has worked with is violinist Yehudi Menuhin, who has frequently spoken of the enormous benefits he derived from these physical and mental exercises.

The following morning I visited Yogi Vithaldas in his Manhattan apartment. The simple furnishings had an air of serenity reflecting the man himself.

'Namaste,' he greeted me, bowing in the graceful gesture of palm pressed to palm and lifted to touch the forehead. His years of living away from his home in India had not altered his manner of dress. He wore the traditional *dhoti*, a garment of long narrow white muslin wrapped around his thighs and loins. His strong frame was covered with a loose white embroidered shirt. A bright orange turban framed his face. His dark, smiling eyes shone as he said, 'Come, sit down. Have a cup of tea with me so we can talk.' He had a soft way with words and

18

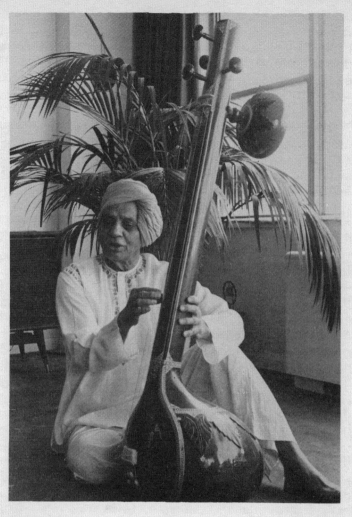

Yogi Vithaldas, a pioneer of yoga in the western world, lives in New York City and, at seventy-two, still teaches the physical and mental disciplines of this centuries-old science. 'When the muscles are properly tuned,' he has said, 'they become resilient and harmonious as the plucked strings of a tambura. We must accept life's inevitable changes by allowing our thoughts to form new patterns with a mind that is flexible and broad in its horizon. If the mind and body are permitted to be idle, degeneration begins.'

spoke with a musical lilt.

I found myself describing in detail the suffering I had gone through for so many years. I told him that the doctors had warned me about the possible danger of ending up in a wheelchair if I overtaxed my spine. He listened attentively, his sallow face calm. From time to time he nodded his head.

After putting me through a series of movements to assess which joints had lost their range of flexibility, he gave me hope. 'Miracles can't happen overnight,' he said, 'but you can get better day by day through your body's own healing powers if you exercise to strengthen your muscles and limber your joints.' His voice rose abruptly when he talked about the excessive use of drugs in the United States. 'Turn on the television and you'll become familiar with all the new drugs that make false promises to relieve a headache, cure a cold, banish tension, insomnia, depression, and what not! Drugs of this kind can be extremely dangerous if the body is not given a chance to heal itself. It will become weakened and dependent on drugs.

'Most people in the western world don't understand nature's healing powers. This is what yoga is all about. It has absolutely nothing to do with religion or mysticism as some people believe. The very word "yoga" comes from the Sanskrit root yuj, "to join." It is the joining of the body and mind to function as one.'

Yogi was a paragon of fitness for a man in his late fifties. He had the grace of an acrobat when he stretched, twisted, and bent his lean, well-toned body. 'If it is given good care, the human body does not have to age as one grows older,' he said. 'Also, the mind will continue to focus sharply if it is well exercised with deep-breathing and mind-control disciplines. The trouble with most people is that they are looking for instant peace of mind. You can't storm the gates of serenity. The road is long and winding and it takes energy and determination to get there.'

He became eloquent when he suggested I take a lesson

from nature to enlarge the boundaries of my thoughts. 'Look at the great blue sky. Its expansiveness does not resist the constant changing of cloud patterns. Think of these clouds as your thoughts, and yourself as the clear blue sky. The sky does not resist the clouds, so you should accept life's inevitable changes by allowing your thoughts to form new patterns with a mind that is flexible and broad in its horizon.'

As I write this story, I have a vivid image of Yogi picking up his tambura and holding upright the long neck of this Asian lute. He plucked the resilent strings in the sounds of a pleasing melody. Then, putting the instrument down, he said: 'When your muscles are properly tuned they will play like the strings of the tambura.' (I have recaptured this image of Yogi Vithaldas, now in his seventies, in a recent photo. See page 19.)

It was an inspiring visit. I left feeling buoyant and restored. With unfailing determination I followed the daily exercises he gave me. There were times when even the most gentle movement was painful. My body rebelled but my spirit was relentless. I knew that the only hope for relief was to keep moving my joints through various stretching exercises. Gradual changes began to happen. I found myself walking with a springier step. The aches that had plagued me for years decreased steadily. This miracle took place in a matter of months. Never had I felt so well and triumphant in my life.

Now, in my fifties, I am free of that chronic nagging pain, though the physical ravages inflicted on my spine are irreversible. Taking care of myself has made the difference between constant pain and a feeling of well-being. Stiffness has given way to agility, weakness to strength. I have learned to respond to my body's signals. There are days when it tells me to continue my exercise a little longer, others when it indicates that it needs complete rest to recharge its energies. I listen.

Through daily meditation I have become attuned to the rhythm of my breath, to the flow of my thoughts, to a growing inner awareness. The depression I had lived with for so many years has faded. A more graceful, reflective attitude with a measure of calm has settled within me which others seem to notice. Recently I spent some time with the Maasai, an East African tribe about whom I was writing a book. After several visits to one of their mud hut villages with my co-author, an English-educated Maasai, the people came to know me. One day the tribal elder decided I should have a Maasai name. Without hesitation he called me *Naserian*, 'the peaceful one.'

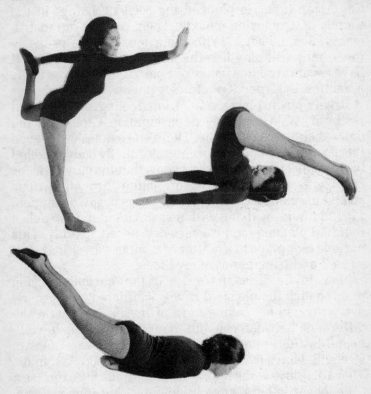

These recent pictures of Rachel Carr show what daily exercise can do. Stiffness gives way to flexibility, weakness to strength. The body becomes supple and strong. Fitness has a way of making time stand still.

Much attention is being drawn to the holistic approach to health, in which the mind is called upon to assist in the healing of the body. Curiously, behind the effectiveness of holistic medicine is the basic theory of yoga that has survived for over four thousand years. It appeals to any society. I have used this theory in natural therapy and have taught it to people of all ages. Some of the most gratifying experiences I have had were with the elderly, who are not likely to reject a new experience if it means hope

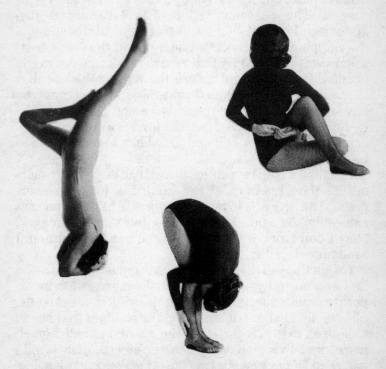

for them. An eighty-year-old lady with advanced rheumatoid arthritis was eager to learn how she could make peace with this crippling disease.

'I know I won't get well,' she told me, 'but at least I want to be able to live out the rest of my life with as little drugs as possible. My dear doctor gives me a pill for depression, another for pain, another for sleep, and so on. Look at the bottles on my dresser!'

Her determination to get better was strong. Though her progress was slow, often agonizing, she looked forward to quiet periods of deep breathing and meditation. The stretching exercises gave her some flexibility in her fingers, and she was able to walk a little more easily with the help of her cane. Changes reflecting an inner calm soon became evident in her life. In her bedroom, bright chintz curtains replaced heavy dark-blue velvet drapes. The pervasive odor of a long illness disappeared. Fresh flowers and bottles of perfume made their appearance. Next to a neat pile of the latest best-sellers was a small tray that held the essential drugs she needed. One could not ignore the inner radiance that shone through her crippled body. Like many others who have discovered self-healing, she couldn't wait to share it. She said, 'I showed my doctor some of the deep-breathing exercises I do and urged him to teach them to his patients!'

A sculptor in his seventies found time every day to sort out his thoughts in quiet reflection and to do his exercises. 'The arthritis in my neck seems to have eased considerably,' he said. 'My back, too, feels much stronger. Now I can work with greater force and imagination. I really feel terrific.'

I often think of the ninety-six-year-old lady I knew who had an unusually active life, yet she managed to incorporate a daily discipline of exercises into her schedule. She boasted to her friends about the changes that began to happen to her. 'I can enjoy the opera and ballet much more since I've been doing these stretches. Also, I find I can read longer now that my power of concentration has improved with the mind-control exercises I do.'

At one of her dinner parties she told this story to the delight of her guests. 'I was sitting in my bedroom doing one of my morning exercises, the one called Alternate Breathing, when I looked up and saw a window washer on his moving platform staring at me with his mouth wide open. He was probably trying to figure out what in the name of heaven this old lady was doing with her eyes closed, shifting her fingers on her nostrils for so long!'

There are many others I have known through the years who have triumphed over their physical afflictions through sheer willpower.

2 FACTS ABOUT ARTHRITIS

The dictionary describes arthritis as 'inflammation of a joint.' The word is derived from the Greek *arth*, meaning 'joint,' and *itis*, 'inflammation.' Ten percent of the world's population suffers from this crippling disease which attacks infants and elderly people alike. Government surveys conducted in the United States in 1976 reveal these staggering figures:

> Over 30 million Americans are its victims: 16,000,000 people have osteoarthritis; 6,500,000 have rheumatoid arthritis; and 250,000 children are afflicted. Studies show that 97 percent of people over 60 have sufficient arthritis to show up in X-ray films. Fortunately for many, their symptoms are so slight that they cause no problems.*

According to the Arthritis Foundation these sufferers spend almost half a billion dollars a year on worthless, harmful drugs, treatments, and special diets.

There are five common types of arthritis: osteoarthritis, rheumatoid arthritis, lupus, spinal arthritis, and gout.

Osteoarthritis, the most common form, derives its name from the Greek word *osteon*, meaning 'bone.' The -*itis* in the word is a misnomer because little inflamma-

---

*From *Arthritis: The Basic Facts*. Copyright © 1978 by the Arthritis Foundation, Atlanta, Ga.

tion exists in most forms. In this disease there is a combination of cartilage and bony changes, the bony changes often appearing as overgrowth of bony areas in the form of protuberances called *osteophytes*.

Two types of osteoarthritis are recognized, primary and secondary. Frequently, primary osteoarthritis appears in the tip joints of the fingers; the characteristic growth is commonly known as Herberden's Nodes, after the British doctor who first described them. The middle joints of the fingers, the base of the thumb, the hips, the knees, and the upper and lower spine can also be involved. Its appearance in the joints often has a distinctive pattern that is readily recognizable. Primary osteoarthritis is most prevalent in postmenopausal females, and there is an inheritance pattern. The secondary type arises from an injury. The injury may or may not be readily apparent, so the distinction between primary and secondary osteoarthritis is often unclear in a particular patient who may indeed have both types. The pain and immobility can be severe, and gentle exercise to preserve or improve joint action is of the utmost importance.

Rheumatoid arthritis, the most crippling common form, occurs most often in women, especially between the ages of twenty and forty. Early symptoms are soreness, stiffness, and aching in the joints, mostly of the hands and feet. There may be loss of appetite and loss of weight. This inflammatory and chronic disease can affect many other organ systems including the lungs, skin, blood vessels, muscles, heart, and even the eyes.

Rheumatoid arthritis is not directly inherited, but recent research has shown that one can inherit a predisposition to the disease. Blood tests reveal a genetic marker in those likely to become victims when an unknown trigger sets it off.

Victims of rheumatoid arthritis live in constant fear of becoming crippled. It takes a compassionate person to understand the degree of a victim's suffering. The pressure of bed clothing on the skin can become unbearable, and fatigue so intense that it is nauseating. Drug therapy

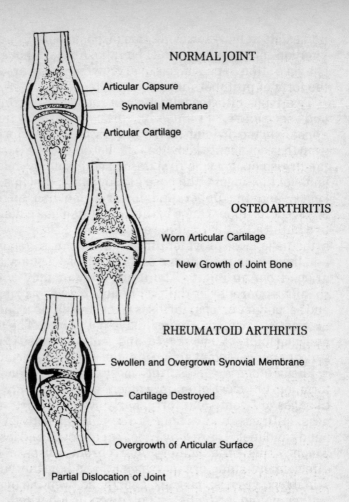

NORMAL JOINT

Articular Capsure
Synovial Membrane
Articular Cartilage

OSTEOARTHRITIS

Worn Articular Cartilage
New Growth of Joint Bone

RHEUMATOID ARTHRITIS

Swollen and Overgrown Synovial Membrane
Cartilage Destroyed
Overgrowth of Articular Surface
Partial Dislocation of Joint

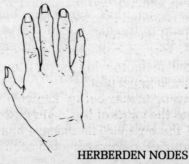

HERBERDEN NODES

28

is essential to help the sufferer physically and mentally. But drugs alone cannot be expected to change a victim's severe mental depression and feeling of futility. Through gentle physical therapy the suffering can be eased, and through therapy of the mind one can make peace with this affliction.

Lupus arthritis is also known as SLE, an abbreviation of its medical name, systemic lupus erythematosis. Lupus, like its cousin rheumatoid arthritis, claims more women than men as its victims. But lupus rarely deforms the bone. When deformity does occur, as in the hands, it is usually caused by slippage of the joints rather than their destruction. It is often the tendons and ligaments around the joints that become loose. In lupus, organs other than the joints are often seriously involved, including the kidneys, skin, blood cells, heart, and lung linings. Factors can usually be found in the victim's blood that cause damage to the body's own tissues, making lupus an 'autoimmune' disease. With the help of drug therapy and physical exercise, the sufferer has a good chance of preserving joint mobility.

Spinal arthritis is the common term for ankylosing spondylitis, meaning 'stiff spine.' While this form of arthritis attacks the spine primarily, it can also attack other joints, especially the weight-bearing joints. Commonly an inherited disease, it usually affects males more seriously than females, and can begin in the late teens and early twenties. In its worst form it can result in a completely stiff spine. With some other spinal diseases it shares a genetic marker called HLA–B27, which can now be revealed in a blood test.

Anti-inflammatory drugs, correct posture, rest, and gentle exercise can aid in preserving mobility of the spine and in decreasing the pain level. Sleeping on a firm mattress is important.

Gouty arthritis, better known as gout, attacks and inflames the joints of the lower extremities, particularly that of the big toe. The disease has been widely known for centuries, having affected such historical figures as

Achilles, Alexander the Great, Kublai Khan, Leonardo da Vinci, Henry VIII, Sir Isaac Newton, Charles Darwin, and Benjamin Franklin (it occurs primarily in men). It was generally believed that gout was caused by over-indulgence in drink, sex, and food. While overindulgence in alcohol can precipitate an attack of gout, the disease is caused by a buildup of uric acid in the blood. The excess uric acid combines with sodium, and the crystal formed settles in the joints and soft tissue where it causes inflammation and extreme pain. Fortunately gout responds to drug therapy. However, if untreated, it can cause a devastating chronic arthritis that can simulate rheumatoid arthritis. In this stage it is important to treat the condition with drugs and with mobility and muscle-toning exercises.

DIET AND ARTHRITIS

Much has been written about nutrition for arthritis. The Arthritis Foundation emphasizes that there is no scientific evidence that specific diets or foods can remedy arthritis, with the exceptions of gout, where over-indulgence in alcohol can trigger an attack. Gout can be controlled with medication and by avoidance of foods high in uric acid, such as liver, pancreas, and brain. Also, drinking a lot of plain water increases urine flow and removes uric acid from the body. In general, of course, a diet is recommended for overweight persons to reduce the burden carried by arthritic joints.

Don't be easily convinced when you hear stories of how some people have been cured of arthritis by taking massive doses of vitamin C, vitamin E, or vitamin B_6, or by avoiding citrus fruits, or by eating two eggs daily. Play it safe. First consult your doctor. He knows your physical condition and what your body may be lacking. A cure for one person may be useless or damaging for another.

The best possible diet for an arthritic condition is wholesome food that includes essential nutrients—

proteins, carbohydrates, fats, vitamins, and minerals—eaten at regular, well-spaced intervals. Raw fruit, leafy vegetables, and whole-grain cereals should be included if you are not allergic to them. Water is without question the body's best purifier. It acts as an excellent laxative. Since the body loses more than a quart of water a day through perspiration and urine, it should be replenished by drinking about two quarts of liquid daily. When the body takes in too little water, waste products are not sufficiently diluted for the kidneys to excrete them. Alcohol can be tolerated by the body only in small amounts. It becomes toxic when taken in excess. Avoid drinking too much coffee or tea. These stimulants can have an adverse effect on the body.

Emotional factors influence a person's eating habits. Lonely people tend to eat a lot to compensate for a feeling of isolation. Boredom is another cause for overeating or nibbling. Weight is easily gained when the foods eaten provide more energy than is needed. Excess food energy is stored in the body as fat. By supplying your body regularly with too much food, you will have an obvious weight gain. If the foods you eat provide less energy than you need, your body uses stored fat.

The unit of food energy is the calorie. If you have the kind of arthritis that restricts your activity, you should cut down on your intake of calories to avoid gaining weight. The only way to maintain ideal weight is to balance the calories provided by food and those used by the body. To lose weight, fewer calories must be consumed than the body uses. It takes about 3,500 extra calories to produce a pound of stored fat. Easy to gain, but hard to lose!

By using some willpower you can maintain your ideal weight. Simply envision yourself as slim and attractive. Every time you are tempted to reach for rich foods, recall that desired image and you will be able to overcome temptation. It is well worth the effort.

Many diet programs concentrate on losing weight rapidly. Once that short-term goal is reached, those who follow such a diet revert to their old eating habits, and before they know it the excess pounds are back. If you plan your meals around lower-calorie foods that you enjoy, it will be much easier to stick to a diet of this kind. Rich meals and highly seasoned foods eaten regularly will load down the system and make it sluggish.

Nervous tension and poor muscular tone of the abdominal muscles can be a cause of a sluggish colon. An excellent way to tone up these muscles is the Abdominal Lift on page 82. In Chapter 4 there are deep-breathing exercises to ease tension and help calm your nerves.

DOES WEATHER AFFECT ARTHRITIS SUFFERERS?

A climate that is generally warm and dry with a relatively stable barometric pressure is ideal for arthritis sufferers. While such a climate cannot cure arthritis, it does contribute to a general feeling of well-being. But it is rarely a sufficient factor to warrant uprooting oneself for a change of residence.

THE DANGERS OF PAIN-KILLING DRUGS

Pain is nature's way of warning that an injured joint or muscle is being overworked, or that the body is in need of rest so it can heal itself. Pain-killing drugs numb the body's sensations. If you are unaware of overexertion because of these drugs, you will push your body too hard and risk fatigue and damage.

HOW MUCH EXERCISE?

This depends on your physical condition. If you listen to your body's signals, you will be able to judge the type of exercises you can safely do. Go slowly at first to build up your stamina and increase your range of flexibility. Exercise each joint gently. Quick, jerky movements can be injurious. Expect temporary setbacks. Aches and pains are bound to develop before the body adjusts to an exercise routine. But when you get a pain signal in a muscle, ligament, or joint, and the pain increases during and after exercise, you are obviously overtaxing that part of your body. Use restraint.

While rest reduces inflammation, too much rest will cause stiffness in the affected joints. Joints must be stretched regularly to maintain their normal range of motion; otherwise they will freeze. Overexercising, however, can cause more pain and quicker freezing.

WHAT EXERCISE CAN DO FOR ARTHRITIS

- Preserves mobility of joints.
- Restores proper circulation essential for the body to carry out its own healing.
- Body excretes less calcium; preserves a sturdier support structure.
- Nourishes cartilage in joints; builds stronger tissues and muscle tone; builds reserve strength.
- Fresh oxygen and nutrients are carried by the bloodstream to all tissues and organs of the body; at the same time toxic waste materials are expelled.
- Induces healthier sleep pattern when the body is well exercised.
- Helps maintain lean body weight.
- Fights depression and anxiety.

3 THE SUPERBLY DESIGNED HUMAN BODY

Thomas Jefferson said, 'In my view no knowledge can be more satisfactory to man than his own frame, its parts, their functions and actions.'

The Greeks and Romans had an esthetic appreciation of the body's form. Sculptors like Michelangelo and Rodin, who studied its inner structure, found it a source of wonder. But most people are quite unaware of the intricacies of the body—as long as their own is running smoothly. The body can take a good deal of abuse, but it will finally rebel when the muscles can no longer function with ease and the body's condition is weakened.

Nature has given only one body to a customer, and it must serve us all our lives. When we hear such alarming statements as 'over 70 million Americans suffer from low back pain,' we begin to wonder why so many people are victims of back trouble. Low back pain is attributed to muscles that have become stiff and short due to lack of exercise. Weak muscles can easily be wrenched by a slightly wrong move or twist. If the wrench is severe enough, it can tear or rupture a ligament, the band of elastic fibrous tissue that connects bone to bone.

When the human body is kept in peak condition, all its parts function in perfect teamwork. The body is superbly rigged. Bone, muscle, and connective tissue are the basic elements of support. Body movement is possible because bones are connected by joints, which in turn are linked by ligaments. Joints of the extremities, such as the hips,

34

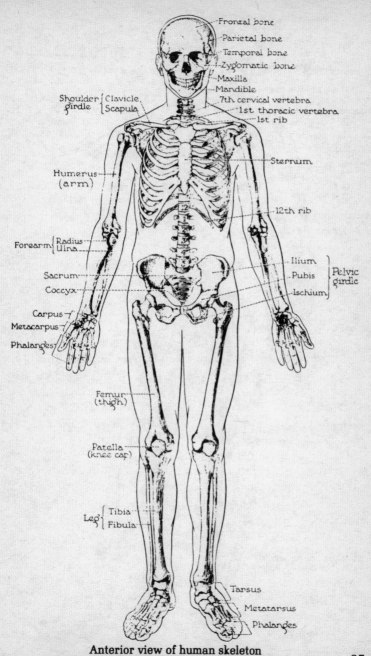

Frontal bone
Parietal bone
Temporal bone
Zygomatic bone
Maxilla
Mandible
7th cervical vertebra
1st thoracic vertebra
1st rib

Shoulder {Clavicle
girdle {Scapula

Sternum

Humerus
(arm)

12th rib

Forearm {Radius
{Ulna

Ilium
Pubis } Pelvic girdle
Ischium

Sacrum
Coccyx

Carpus
Metacarpus
Phalanges

Femur
(thigh)

Patella
(knee cap)

Leg {Tibia
{Fibula

Tarsus
Metatarsus
Phalanges

Anterior view of human skeleton

35

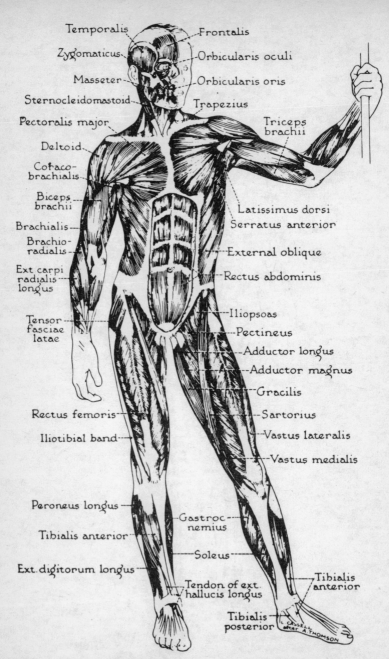

Temporalis
Zygomaticus
Masseter
Sternocleidomastoid
Pectoralis major
Deltoid
Coraco-brachialis
Biceps brachii
Brachialis
Brachio-radialis
Ext carpi radialis longus
Tensor fasciae latae
Rectus femoris
Iliotibial band
Peroneus longus
Tibialis anterior
Ext. digitorum longus

Frontalis
Orbicularis oculi
Orbicularis oris
Trapezius
Triceps brachii
Latissimus dorsi
Serratus anterior
External oblique
Rectus abdominis
Iliopsoas
Pectineus
Adductor longus
Adductor magnus
Gracilis
Sartorius
Vastus lateralis
Vastus medialis
Gastrocnemius
Soleus
Tibialis anterior
Tendon of ext. hallucis longus
Tibialis posterior

L. CASSELL after A. THOMSON

Muscles of the body, anterior view

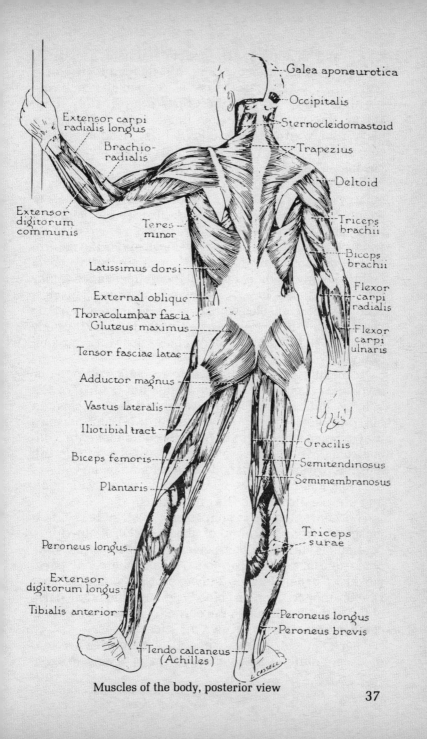

Extensor carpi
radialis longus

Brachio-
radialis

Extensor
digitorum
communis

Teres
minor

Latissimus dorsi

External oblique

Thoracolumbar fascia

Gluteus maximus

Tensor fasciae latae

Adductor magnus

Vastus lateralis

Iliotibial tract

Biceps femoris

Plantaris

Peroneus longus

Extensor
digitorum longus

Tibialis anterior

Tendo calcaneus
(Achilles)

Galea aponeurotica

Occipitalis

Sternocleidomastoid

Trapezius

Deltoid

Triceps
brachii

Biceps
brachii

Flexor
carpi
radialis

Flexor
carpi
ulnaris

Gracilis

Semitendinosus

Semimembranosus

Triceps
surae

Peroneus longus
Peroneus brevis

Muscles of the body, posterior view

37

knees, and shoulders, are flexible and move freely. To reduce friction in movement, these joints are lined with cartilage, a smooth tissue. A special membrane that lines the joint cavity secretes a lubricating fluid. When the joints lack this fluid, they rub against each other, creating friction. This grinding action causes the area around the damaged bony structure to become inflamed.

Skeletal muscles act as cables, pulling on the joints to make possible a variety of movement. The bones to which they are attached act as levers, the joints as fulcrums. Skeletal muscles are often referred to as voluntary muscles because they move under the control of the will; however, they also take part in reflex movements. Owing to their cross-striped appearance under the microscope, they are known as striated muscles. Many skeletal muscles work in pairs. When one of a pair contracts, the other relaxes, setting that part of the body in motion. In fact, the majority of muscles work in group action.

According to traditional western science, smooth, or involuntary, muscles are not under the control of the will, but Indian yogis have proved that these muscles *can be controlled*. These are the visceral (organ) muscles that receive their signals from the autonomic, or self-controlled, nervous system. The fibers of smooth muscles are spindle shaped and are found in the walls of the stomach, intestines, blood vessels, urinary bladder, and uterus; also in the iris and eyelids.

The heart, which is shaped like a strawberry, is a muscular organ made up of striated fibers joined in a continuous network. It receives signals from the autonomic nervous system, although it has an internal 'pacemaker.' The heart needs daily exercise. When the heart rate is stepped up, more blood is pumped to other parts of the body, and through the coronary arteries and their smaller branches, to its own muscular tissues.

There is never a time when all the muscles are in a quiescent state. It takes energy to move a muscle, even the slightest effort, as in grasping a feather. When we lift a pencil, turn the head, or carry something, the muscles in action become tense. They shorten and tighten, regardless of the weight they are bearing. When a muscle is not in use, it returns to its normal length and relaxes. A muscle that is dormant becomes tight, tense, and weak. A tight muscle creates chronic tension, which prohibits muscular relaxation. A muscle must be able to relax; that is part of its function. Muscles that are exercised regularly require more oxygen from the bloodstream to maintain their stretch, suppleness, and resilience.

The charts on pages 35, 36, and 37 give you a clear understanding of how the skeletal and muscular systems are constructed.

4 DEEP BREATHING: THE ELIXIR OF LIFE

Breathing is so natural that most of us don't realize how important it is to breathe properly. Our mental energy is stepped up when the brain gets a healthy supply of oxygen. As the bloodstream is infused with oxygen, cells are revitalized. A reservoir of energy is built up. This increases the body's recuperative powers, helps to calm the nerves, induces restful sleep, and slows down the aging process.

An interesting experiment was devised in 1969 by clinical psychologists at the Veterans Administration Hospital in Buffalo, New York.* Thirteen elderly men were placed in a pressurized chamber and exposed intermittently to 100 percent oxygen. After two treatments daily for fifteen days the patients showed as much as 25 percent increase on the standard memory tests. The oxygen treatment had stimulated their brain cells and increased their vitality. The same results can be brought about much more simply by increasing the oxygen supply to the brain through deep-breathing exercises.

Doctors who are familiar with yoga breathing have borrowed these scientific techniques to treat their patients for depression, nervous tension, and insomnia,

*Eleanor A. Jacobs, Ph.D., Peter W. Winter, M.D., Harry J. Alvis, M.D., and S. Mouchly Small, M.D. 'Hyperbaric Oxygen Effect on Cognition and Behavior in the Aged,' reprinted from Jules H. Masserman, M.D., ed. *Current Psychiatric Therapies*, Vol. II. (New York, Grune & Stratton, 1971.)

and have adapted them for natural childbirth. People with respiratory ailments such as bronchial asthma and emphysema can be helped by the long drawn-out breathing vibrations produced during yoga breathing; the stamina of the lungs is increased and muscle tension is reduced. Smokers suffering from shortness of breath can clear their lungs of congestion through deep breathing; some even lose their desire to smoke.

Since the autonomic nervous system controls breathing, any state of emotional stress—fear, anger, excitement—will make you breathe faster and will accelerate your heartbeat. To compensate for a greater physical effort, your lungs take in more oxygen. Once you are aware of what stress can do to your body, you can control your emotions to some degree during psychologically tense situations by using deep-breathing techniques.

Nature intended us to breathe deeply, filling the lungs with air. The lungs are large spongy organs with thin walls. Oxygen is absorbed through the walls of the lungs, then carried by the bloodstream to all the cells of the body. During exhalation, the lungs expel carbon dioxide, a waste material from the cells that is picked up by the blood.

There are several reasons why we should breathe through the nostrils rather than through the mouth. First, the air-cleaning process for the lungs begins in the nose, the hairs acting as filters for dust particles. Second, air passing through the nose is warmed and moistened. Third, when we breathe out through the nostrils rather than the mouth, the lungs are strengthened since they take longer to deflate. However, there are times, such as in brisk walking or running, when exhaling through the mouth is desirable for a quicker supply of oxygen.

It is much easier to inhale deeply than to exhale; that is why breathing exercises emphasize prolonged exhalations, usually in a ratio to inhalation of two to one (twice as long). Singers know this. The breath is strengthened and its duration increased with concentration on the slow expulsion of air from the lungs.

You can test the strength of your lungs by trying to blow out a candle held eight inches or so away, or by inflating a balloon or a paper bag. If the lungs are weak, you will have trouble blowing out the flame or you will quickly run out of breath. Whatever the condition of your lungs, they will be greatly strengthened by the deep-breathing exercises given in this chapter.

Practice each breathing exercise slowly and faithfully until you become familiar with it. Then do three or four different breathing patterns each day to fully derive their benefits. Vary the exercises every so often.

THREE BASIC BREATHING EXERCISES

Practice these breathing techniques that appear on pages 43 to 47 every day for three weeks so you will become familiar with their individual patterns and benefits:

Abdominal Breathing exercises the diaphragm, abdomen, and lower lobes of the lungs.

Rib-Cage Breathing exercises the pectoral (chest) muscles and the middle parts of the lungs.

Complete Breathing exercises the lower, middle, and uppermost parts of the lungs.

It is easy to remember the key to correct breathing:

Inhale and expand the abdomen.
Exhale and contract the abdomen.

ABDOMINAL BREATHING

Lie on your back, knees bent. Place one hand on the abdomen to feel the movement of the diaphragm. This principal muscle in breathing is dome shaped, and separates the chest from the abdomen.

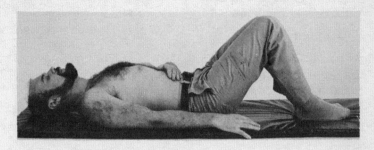

Close your eyes. Inhale through the nostrils (mouth closed). Feel the abdomen expanding. Keep the chest still.

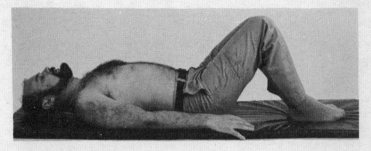

Exhale through the nostrils (mouth closed). Feel the abdomen contracting.

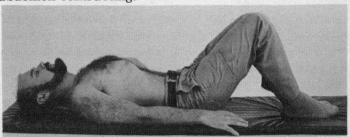

Practice this technique while concentrating on the rise and fall of your abdomen. Keep your chest as still as possible.

Repeat ten times without stopping, following this ratio:

Inhale to the count of five seconds.
Exhale to the count of five seconds.

Gradually increase the ratio until you are able to follow this rhythm:

Inhale to the count of five seconds.
Exhale to the count of ten seconds.

Abdominal breathing, when practiced properly, can have a calming influence on your mind and body.

RIB-CAGE BREATHING

This breathing technique can be done standing or sitting.

Place your hands on the rib cage. Inhale. Feel the rib cage moving out and the chest expanding.

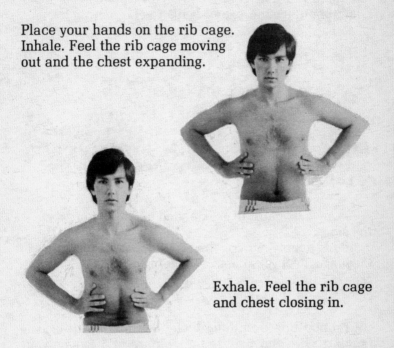

Exhale. Feel the rib cage and chest closing in.

Practice this technique while concentrating on the movement of your rib cage: moving out and closing in.

Repeat ten times without stopping, following this ratio:

Inhale to the count of five seconds.
Exhale to the count of five seconds.

Gradually increase the ratio until you are able to follow this rhythm:

Inhale to the count of five seconds.
Exhale to the count of ten seconds.

COMPLETE BREATHING

In this breathing technique the flow of your breath is like water poured into a pitcher: first the bottom, then the middle, and finally the top. When emptying, the top is first, then the middle, and lastly the bottom.

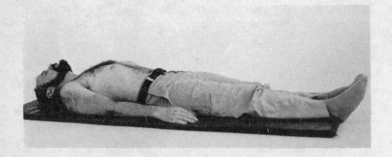

Lie on your back, legs extended and together, arms at the sides.

Inhale deeply, pulling the air into the topmost parts of the lungs. Feel your chest expanding and your shoulders rising. Exhale, slowly releasing the air until the chest is relaxed and the abdomen sinks in toward the spine.

Practice this breathing technique until you become familiar with the way the air enters and leaves your lungs. There should be a rhythm in the breathing. Follow this ratio:

Inhale to the count of five seconds.
Exhale to the count of ten seconds.

Repeat ten times without stopping.

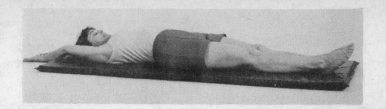

This is the second step to complete breathing. While on your back with arms at your sides and legs together, inhale deeply. At the same time stretch your arms overhead until the backs of your hands are touching the floor, or as far down as you can. You will notice that this action pulls in your abdomen as the air is drawn up into the topmost part of your lungs. Hold your breath and stretch from head to toe. Then exhale and slowly raise your arms forward and down without resistance. Your abdomen will gradually sink in toward the spine.

Practice these movements first, then follow this ratio:

Inhale to the count of five seconds.
Hold your breath for ten seconds.
Exhale for ten seconds.

Repeat ten times without stopping. If you feel lightheaded, it is because of hyperventilation. Rest a moment and it will disappear.

This breathing technique must not be done mechanically. Your mind is held quietly in control. As you inhale, feel the flow of energy entering your body. While holding your breath and stretching, allow the energy to reach its peak. Then as you exhale, feel tension knots slowly dissolving.

You can also do this breathing exercise sitting or standing. It will pick up your energy and release tension.

RESISTANCE BREATHING

The exercises on pages 49 and 50, done while sitting, will strengthen the lungs and tone muscles in the chest and arms. By tensing your arm and shoulder muscles to resist the movement, you are pitting one muscle against the other. This should be done three times for fifteen counts without stopping.

If your lungs are not strong enough for this retention, then build your resistance gradually. Hold your breath for five counts, then ten, and finally increase it to fifteen. In a short time, your lungs will gain stamina and you will be able to do these exercises with ease.

HORIZONTAL STRETCH

Sit with hands clasped close to the chest. Inhale deeply.
Hold your breath as you stretch the arms forward. Use
resistance to pull the arms toward you, touching the
chest. Do this three times without stopping while holding
the breath. Each movement takes five seconds. Exhale
and relax. Repeat three times.

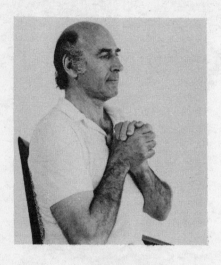

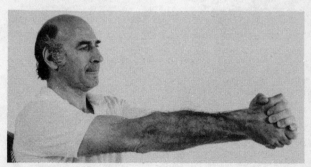

VERTICAL STRETCH

Sit with hands clasped behind the head. Inhale deeply. Hold your breath as you stretch the arms upward. Use resistance to pull the arms down behind your head, touching the back of the neck. Do this three times without stopping while holding the breath. Each movement takes five seconds. Exhale and relax. Repeat three times.

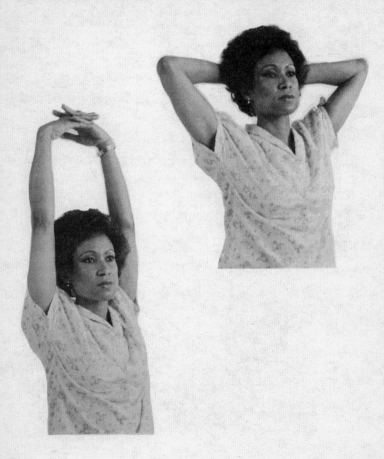

BELLOWS BREATH

Acting as a bellows, this effective breathing exercise pumps energy into the lungs in a brisk rhythm. It is also called Runner's Breath because the lungs are exerted to their utmost, as in running. This exercise benefits the nervous, circulatory, and digestive systems.

Too many words used to describe this breathing pattern will make it sound more difficult than it actually is. Just remember that as you exhale forcefully through your nostrils, the sound should be like quick outward sniffs in a staccato rhythm. Don't make any effort to inhale. Inhalation is a natural reaction. If you inhale consciously you will destroy the rhythm of the forceful outward breaths.

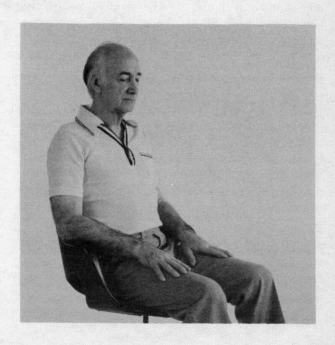

Sit with your eyes closed. Keep your hands on your lap, fingers loosely cupped.

Exhale forcefully through your nostrils; at the same time contract your abdomen to expel air. There should be a powerful push from your diaphragm and a thrust from your throat. *Without stopping*, release the contraction and your lungs will automatically take in air.

Practice slowly to build up an even rhythm. It should sound like the tick of a clock, keeping a steady beat. Repeat this rhythm up to the count of ten, then stop. Inhale deeply and relax before practicing again.

Don't try to build up the expulsions until you have mastered ten counts easily. Once you can do this, you will be able to do from 50 to 100 expulsions with ease. It will give you a marvelous sensation of energy surging through your body. At the same time its therapeutic effects will get rid of a headache caused by tension and pick up sagging energy.

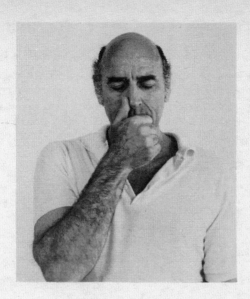

ALTERNATE BREATHING

This dynamic exercise of breathing through alternate nostrils can quiet the mind and relieve tension when done with full concentration. It has other benefits. If your nostrils are blocked, press your right thumb on the right nostril, then forcibly inhale and exhale through the left nostril ten to fifteen times. Repeat the same forceful breathing through the right nostril. It will cure a headache and relieve a sinus attack.

Here is the finger pattern for one round of alternate breathing:

Place the right thumb on the right nostril, index and middle fingers turned in, the fourth and little fingers held near the left nostril.

Press on right nostril with thumb. Inhale to the count of five seconds through the left nostril.

Close the left nostril with the fourth finger. Release the right nostril, and exhale to the count of ten seconds.

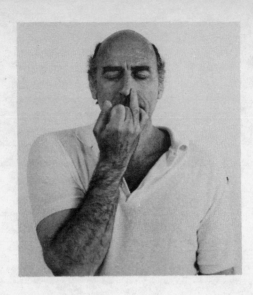

Without stopping, inhale again through the right nostril to the count of five seconds.

Close that nostril with the thumb. Release the left nostril and exhale completely to the count of ten seconds.

Allow your breath to flow continuously from one nostril to the other without staggering. Think of your breath rising and falling with a musical cadence. Feel its rhythm with your mind and your body.

When you have learned the technique of alternate breathing, follow this ratio to do one round:

Inhale to the count of five seconds.
Exhale to the count of ten seconds.
Inhale to the count of five seconds.
Exhale to the count of ten seconds.

Repeat for three rounds without stopping.

5 YOUR MIND CAN HELP HEAL YOUR BODY

One of the most inspiring stories about self-healing is told by Norman Cousins in his book *Anatomy of an Illness*. His description of his recovery from a crippling, supposedly irreversible disease gives hope to the seriously ill. He wrote, 'It all began when I said I decided that some experts don't really know enough to make a pronouncement of doom on a human being. And I said I hoped they would be careful about what they said to others; they might be believed and that could be the beginning of the end. . . . If negative thinking can affect the body and mind, why can't positive thinking act as a reversal? I have learned never to underestimate the capacity of the human mind and body to regenerate, even when the prospects seem wretched. The life-force may be the least understood force on earth.'

The yogis, who are masters of understanding the human mind and body and its capabilities, call this life-force *prana*. It is the source of a power that we can draw from within once we know how to tap it. It can bring calmness and balance in our lives. It can refresh and revitalize the spirit.

When we are able to understand the workings of the mind we realize how restless it can be. Without controls, it may run amok, and when overwhelmed by negative thoughts, become so depressed that we are unable to function. By turning to 'miracle' mood drugs to relieve that depression, we get only temporary relief. Furthermore, when the mind is sedated, the senses become dulled.

The mind-control exercises in this chapter will help you direct your thoughts and bring your mind under quiet control. As your mind becomes more orderly, you will gain a better insight into yourself, and you will be able to discard negative influences. You will be amazed at the results you can achieve through the power of your mind. It can help heal your body and give you a source of energy you never knew you had.

If the idea of mind control is new to you and you are uncertain about the benefits of this type of exercise, I suggest that you pick out the one that appeals to you the most and give it a try. Do the exercise for just a few minutes a day for about a week. With each day your ability to sit quietly and concentrate will increase immeasurably. Simply sitting still reflects stillness within.

You have probably heard a great deal about meditation. Meditation in practice is neither mystical nor highly intellectual. Anyone can learn to do it. Meditation may be thought of simply as a clearinghouse to help sort out the essential from the nonessential. It may also be considered as a controlled process of uniting body and mind so they can respond and become attuned to one another. All the mind-control exercises described here have much in common with meditation.

The way you sit when you meditate or do these exercises is important. Sit with your spine resting comfortably against the back of a chair with your legs uncrossed, or sit cross-legged on a rug. A sitting position will keep you from falling into a sleep stage. Be sure that your back and head are in a straight line, but not held rigidly. To prevent fidgeting, let your hands rest limply on your knees, or keep your fingers loosely interlocked. Then close your eyes lightly.

No one can tell you how long you should meditate. Ten minutes a day will help enormously. How will you know when the time is up? It is most disturbing to have a timer ticking away while you are trying to turn your mind inward. The best solution is to *feel* the amount of time you need for each day. It could be five minutes, ten minutes, fifteen minutes, or even twenty minutes.

To prevent the monotony of practicing the same mental exercise every day, you can vary the disciplines from time to time.

CANDLE CONCENTRATION

This mind-sharpening exercise is done in a dark room so that the candle flame will not lose its luminous quality.

Sit with the candle in easy viewing distance. Gaze at the flame until your eyes begin to tear. It takes from twenty to thirty seconds, depending on the sensitivity of your eyes to light. Blow out the candle and close your eyes. You will see the glow of the flame in full view. It will be bright. Hold on to this image and observe how it changes shape and degree of brightness. It will recede into the distance and become elongated. A black halo with a dotted flame in the center will appear and reappear, then gradually disappear until you lose the image completely.

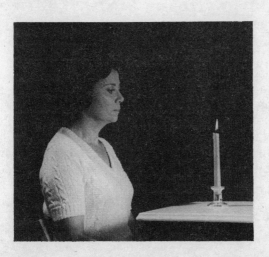

Light the candle again and repeat this exercise three times. You will find that you can hold the image longer in your mind's eye with each practice. Perform this exercise for five minutes every day for a week. There will be a remarkable difference in your powers of concentration and observation. You will gain a strong mental image of the orange-colored flame and the textural quality of the candle itself. You will also notice that the flame has a calming influence on your mind.

NUMERAL CONCENTRATION

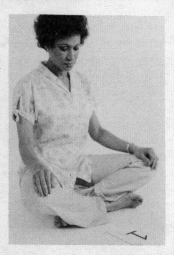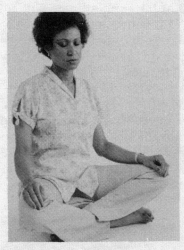

Visualizing a number and concentrating on it as you inhale and exhale deeply will help harness your mind to focus on one thought at a time.

To help you hold the numeral images, write each number on a 4″ × 5″ card in thick black strokes. Place the cards in sequence, in a pile, in front of you as you sit in any comfortable position. Inhale deeply and concentrate on the number 1. Then close your eyes, and in your mind's eye visualize that number. Exhale and open your eyes. Continue this mental exercise until you have reached the number 10. Then reverse the numbers from

10 to 1 in the same way.

As your power of concentration develops, you will be able to do the numeral concentration without looking at the visuals. Start by breathing quietly for a few seconds to establish a calm attitude. Then begin the numeral concentration. Inhale deeply as you count 1. In your mind's eye outline that number and repeat it silently. See it large and clear. Hold the image until you exhale slowly. Inhale again, count 2. Repeat until you reach the number 10. Then begin to count down, starting from 10 to 1. If your mind strays, gently coax it back to the numbers.

YOUR MIND IS A BLACKBOARD

This mental exercise is one of the most effective techniques to bring the mind under quiet control so you can direct its energies successfully.

Take a moment to watch the workings of your mind. Sit still with your eyes closed. Observe how your thoughts skip and hop about like a frisky monkey, without rhyme or reason. If you allow this mental process to continue, you will soon be exhausted. This is precisely what happens to those of us who are unable to control the wanderings of the mind, particularly when it is obsessed with negative and depressing thoughts. We become prisoners of ourselves.

To practice the 'blackboard' technique, sit comfortably in a chair with your back straight. Your feet should rest evenly on the floor, preferably without shoes, and your hands should be placed limply in your lap. Begin to breathe quietly with your eyes closed. Take long, slow, deep breaths to help turn your mind inward. Continue to breathe this way. As your thoughts begin to appear, gently coax them away by wiping the blackboard clean. Repeat this exercise several times and random thoughts will appear with less frequency.

Spend five minutes a day with this mental exercise. In

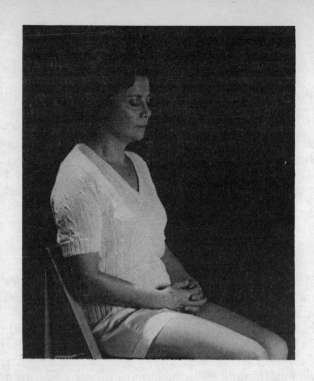

a week or so you will notice changes. Your mind can find moments of rest from its ceaseless wanderings. A wonderful feeling of inner calm will take over. As you continue to meditate daily you will be able to free your mind of the heavy load that negative thinking imposes on it, and you will gain a sense of inner-directed energy that leads to positive action.

HOW TO GET A GOOD NIGHT'S SLEEP

If you are a light or restless sleeper, try these helpful ways to release the anxiety and tension that rob you of sound sleep.

Before turning off the light, be sure the bedroom is well ventilated. An overheated room will dry up the mucous membranes in your nostrils and throat, and give you a stuffy head. Your bedclothes should be light and loose.

Lie stretched out in bed, arms resting loosely at your sides. Tuck a large soft pillow under the knees and a thin soft one under the head so your neck will relax more easily.

As you become more aware of your physical self you will be able to control deeper parts of your body and feel tranquility. Begin by coaxing your muscles into relaxing. Breathe quietly and deeply with your eyes closed.

Stretch your right leg. Pull slowly on your hip and lower back muscles. Keep the rest of your body still. Repeat with the left leg.

Stretch your lower left side, starting with the waist, small of the back, hip, leg, down to the toes. Repeat with the right side.

Stretch upward on the left side, starting with your waist, chest, arms, and fingertips. Repeat with the right side.

Stretch your neck gently, turning the head to the right side, then to the left, and back to its normal position. Feel tense muscles releasing in your face and along the back of the neck. Feel it with your mind, and your body will respond.

Think of waves of relaxation spreading through your feet, legs, abdomen, chest, arms, hands, then along the spine to the small of the back and the buttocks. Let that feeling of relaxation spread to every part of your body.

Continue to breathe deeply and quietly as you listen to the soft signals of your body, to the rhythm of your breath, and to your heart beating.

Yawn and stretch. Talk to your mind. Tell it to be still. Say to it, 'I am tired. I want to sleep now.' Repeat these phrases over and over until you feel the tension flowing out of muscle after muscle. You will begin to experience a state of weightlessness as you fall into the depths of sound sleep.

As you practice it will gradually become easier to feel total relaxation of body and mind.

6 EXERCISING THE BODY

SOME HELPFUL TIPS

SOME HELPFUL TIPS

Do all the exercises slowly and smoothly while breathing calmly.

- For exercises performed in a lying position, use a padded mat, folded blanket, or a towel over a rug. Some of these exercises can be done in bed if your mattress is very firm.
- Wear light stretch clothes when you exercise.
- Never exercise on a full stomach. Wait at least an hour after you have eaten so as not to disturb the digestive system.
- To combat morning stiffness, take a hot shower or bath before exercising. Allow the heat to penetrate sore muscles and joints.
- Take it easy if your joints are inflamed. Exercise them gently. Even the slightest movement of painful joints will protect them from becoming 'frozen.' When the inflammation subsides you will be able to move your joints more easily.

By making exercise habit-forming, you can undo years of neglect and banish unnecessary suffering.

SPINE, ABDOMEN, AND BUTTOCKS

HOW TO KEEP YOUR BACK IN SHAPE

Your spine is a marvel of engineering. Composed of vertebrae, or bony rings, it curves like a question mark; a mass of cables resembling a switchboard links the brain and spinal cord with other parts of the body. Its flexibility enables it to twist, bend, and absorb shocks. The backbone consists of three groups of vertebrae—the cervical, thoracic, lumbar—followed by the sacrum and coccyx. Each pair of vertebrae is equipped with cushioning discs that act as shock absorbers between the vertebrae. A disc is made up of semielastic casing and a gelatinous center, and any stress inflicted on the back is transmitted directly to it. The discs are constantly exposed to injuries, some serious, requiring surgery, others less so but painful all the same, when the injured disc presses on the nerve. The irritated nerve will, in turn, throw one of its muscles into a spasm. The overtaxed muscle becomes a hard knotty mass. If the sciatic nerve is affected, any movement, no matter how slight, becomes torturous.

A common ailment is backache, frequently caused by a sedentary life. If you sit for long periods at a time without exercising, the chances are that your back is vulnerable to injury. Even the slightest movement, such as sneezing, can create a painful muscle spasm. A weak back is certain to turn your life into continual misery unless you do something about it.

It may surprise you to know that sitting puts greater pressure on the spine than standing. When you sit, the abdominal muscles that support your back become slack and thrust their portion of the load onto the back muscles. Under such an additional load, the back muscles will slump from fatigue. When strained beyond their limit, they rebel.

People who suffer from chronic back pain should be

aware that emotional stress can increase pain. As muscle tension grows, the pain cycle is aggravated. While heat treatments can relieve pain temporarily, exercise is the best therapy. It will increase blood flow and relieve muscle tension.

You can ease back pain by sleeping on a firm mattress, or with a board placed under a soft one, to give your back good support. A comfortable position for sleeping on your side is to keep your hips and knees flexed, with one leg drawn up slightly. A soft pillow between the knees helps to lessen back pain. When lying on your back, place a soft pillow under the knees, so the knees and hips will be slightly flexed.

If you want permanent relief from low back pain, your spine must be protected by strengthening the muscles that support it. The abdominal musculature is the main support of the back, aided by the gluteals, the muscles you sit on. In the following pages there are helpful tips to relieve back pain and exercises designed to strengthen the supporting muscles so they can carry their own load.

The Right Posture: Standing

If you have a tendency
to slump or stand
swaybacked, your muscles
are weak. Though it may
seem to take less muscle
power to stand this
way, such a stance puts
stress on the back muscles,
throwing them out of kilter.

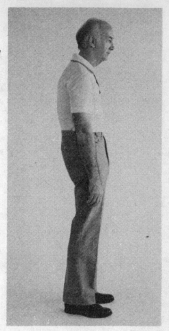

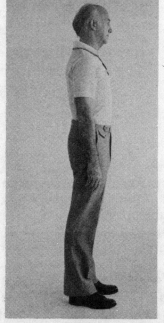

The correct posture is to
stand comfortably with the
buttocks tucked in. Simply
tightening the muscles in the
buttocks now and then will
help to improve your posture.

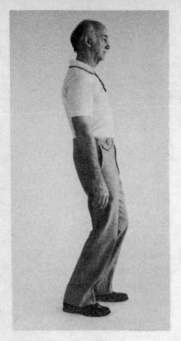

You can relieve muscle fatigue by standing with one foot in front of the other, knees slightly flexed, or by standing with one foot on a raised surface.

The Right Posture: Sitting

Slumping in a chair puts too much weight on the spine and can cause pain in the coccyx (tip of the spine). Since sitting happens to be one of the worst positions for the back, sit in a chair with firm support. Keep your feet on the same level. When you are driving for long periods at a time, stop to stretch and walk around. It will relieve strain on the lower back.

If your life is sedentary, sit in a straight-backed chair with your knees brought up higher than the hips by resting your feet on a stool.

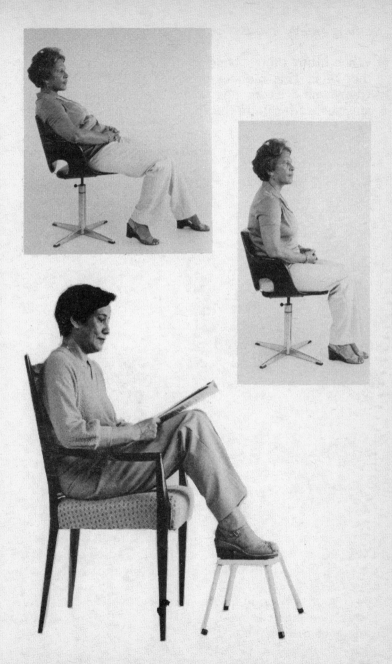

Lifting Heavy Loads

When lifting things, bend from the knees and not from the waist. This reduces pressure on the lumbar area where most backaches occur. Let the powerful leg muscles, rather than the spine, carry the weight of the load.

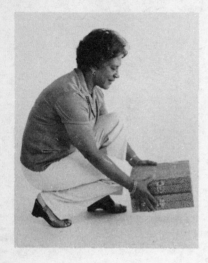

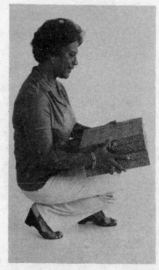

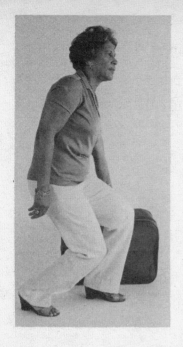

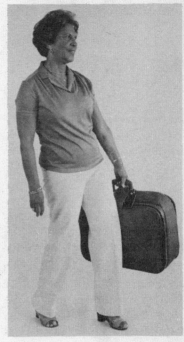

Wearing the Right Kind of Shoes

Women are victims of stylish shoes that contribute to
back problems and leg cramps. Pointed, narrow shoes
pinch the feet, constrict the toes, cause corns, and chafe
the heels. High heels throw the spine out of balance and
thrust the pelvis forward. Wide, flat, ill-fitting shoes
don't support the arches. When our feet hurt, we hurt all
over.

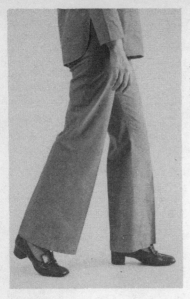

Comfortable shoes with good support and low heels will prevent backaches when you walk or stand for long periods.

RELIEF FOR AN ACHING BACK

Lie on your back with your legs raised, feet resting on a stool or low chair. Keep your arms relaxed at your sides. Close your eyes and remain in this position for at least ten minutes, and the blood will begin to circulate freely. The nagging pain in your back will be eased, and any swelling in your feet will be reduced.

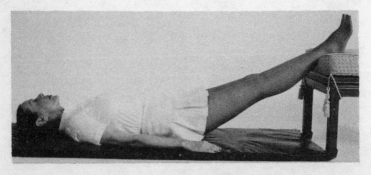

LOWER BACK STRETCH

Lie on your back, knees bent and slightly apart. Interlock fingers and place them on the abdomen. Tighten the buttock muscles and pull in the abdomen at the same time, so the curve of your back will touch the mat. Hold for five counts while breathing deeply. Repeat ten times.

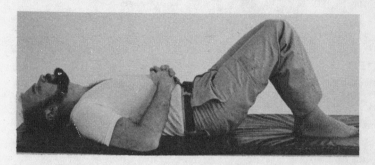

This excellent exercise not only stretches lower back muscles, but also tones up the buttocks and abdomen.

SPINAL STRETCH

In a kneeling position, slide your arms forward until your head touches the mat and arms are stretched out, palms down. Keep your hips above the knees, toes down. Hold for five counts while breathing deeply.

Then slide back to rest on the heels, or as far as you can stretch. Hold for five counts while breathing deeply.

Repeat five times slowly.

These movements will ease tension in the spine and lower back, increasing flexibility at the same time.

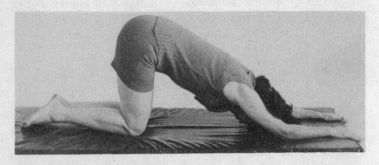

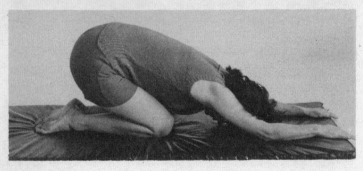

PELVIC STRETCH

Lie on your back, knees bent, feet flat on the floor, and arms at the sides. Inhale, then raise your buttocks as high as you can, putting weight on the shoulders and feet. Breathe freely while slowly raising and lowering the buttocks five times.

When your spine is more limber, rotate the pelvis in a circular motion, ten times toward the right, ten times toward the left. This movement will strengthen and loosen up rigid muscles of the back, pelvis, and hips.

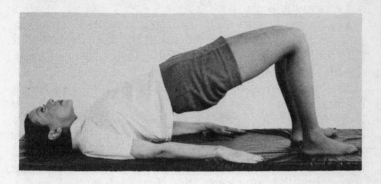

STRENGTHENING THE UPPER ABDOMEN

Fold arms over the chest, or interlock fingers, while stretched out with legs together. Inhale, raise the head slowly, keeping the legs on the mat. Exhale. Hold for ten counts while tightening the abdomen. Lower the head slowly. Repeat five times.

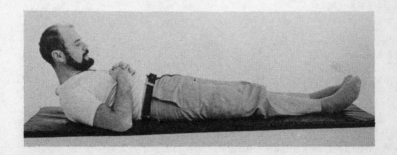

LEG LIFTS

Do each of these three exercises six times, alternating right and left legs. Raise each leg as high as you can without straining.

Lie on back with legs together, arms at your sides, palms down. Inhale, slowly raise left leg. Exhale and hold for five counts while tightening the abdomen. Lower the leg. Repeat with right leg.

Lie face down, arms folded under the forehead, keeping nose clear of the mat. Inhale, slowly raise left leg. Exhale and hold for five counts while tightening the abdomen. Lower the leg. Repeat with the right leg.

These exercises will loosen up the hip flexors and relieve tightness in the lower back, and at the same time strengthen the muscles of the lower abdomen.

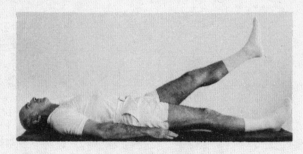

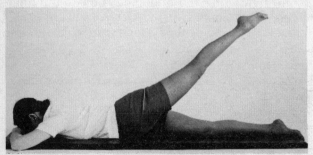

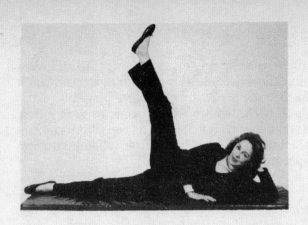

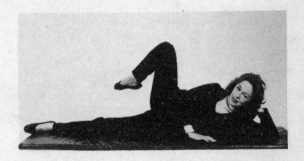

Lie on your left side. Support your head with your left hand, elbow resting on the mat. Place your right hand in front. Raise the right leg as high as you can, keeping it straight. Tense the front and back muscles in the upper leg to exert force without moving the leg. Do this ten times slowly. Then, gently flex and straighten the leg ten times. Keep your back as straight as possible throughout. Repeat on the right side.

This exercise is excellent for the hip flexors and knees, which are weight-bearing joints; it also tones legs, lower back, and abdomen.

SIT-UPS

You can limber your spine and strengthen the abdomen by tightening the muscles as you sit up. Repeat each exercise five times slowly for maximum benefit.

Lie on your back, legs together, arms at your sides. Inhale and stretch arms out in front as you sit up, curving your spine. Exhale. Hold for five counts while tightening the abdomen. Lower your back.

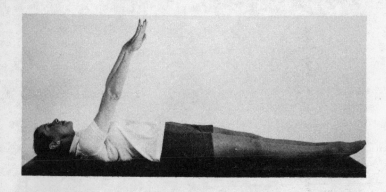

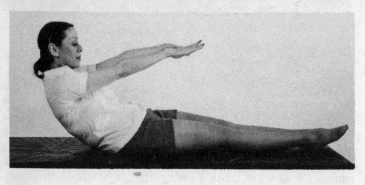

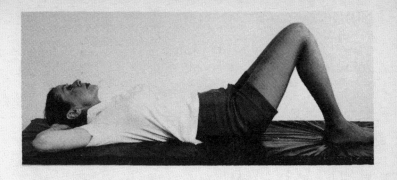

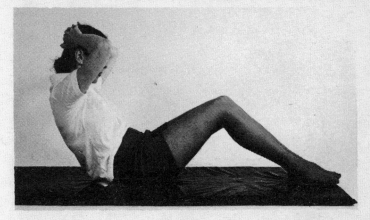

   While on your back, bend your knees, keeping the feet flat and slightly apart. Clasp hands behind your head. Inhale as you sit up, curving your spine. Exhale. Hold for five counts while tightening the abdomen. Lower your back.

LEG ROTATION

There are many benefits to this exercise: leg muscles, spine, and abdomen all get a toning up. It is important to rotate the legs slowly while breathing rhythmically.

Lie on your back, arms at your sides, legs together. Inhale and raise legs, keeping the back on the floor. Breathe freely and rotate legs as if pedaling the wheels of a bicycle. Pedal twenty times slowly.

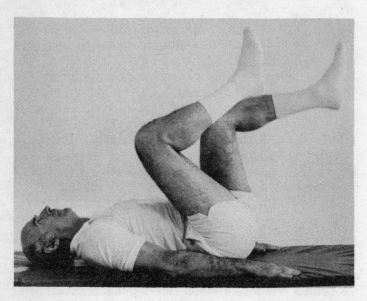

If your back muscles are strong enough, raise your spine, supporting the back with your arms, hands holding the buttocks, and pedal twenty times slowly.

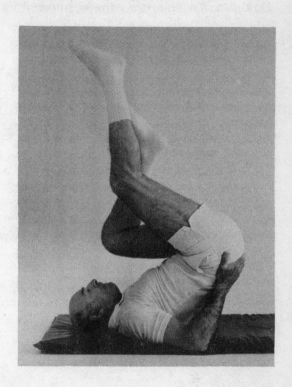

OVERALL FLEXIBILITY

This series will tone and limber the muscles of the lower back and abdomen, and loosen tightness in the hip flexors.

Lie on your back. Bend both knees. Hold the right knee with both hands, pulling toward the chest. Hold for five counts while breathing deeply. Repeat with the left leg. Do these movements six times, alternating the legs.

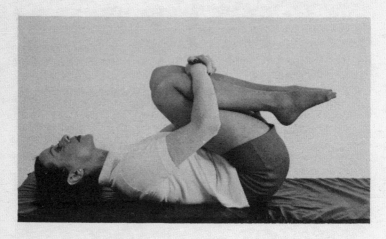

Clasp your hands with fingers interlocked around the knees. Gently press knees toward your chest. Hold for five counts while breathing deeply. Repeat five times.

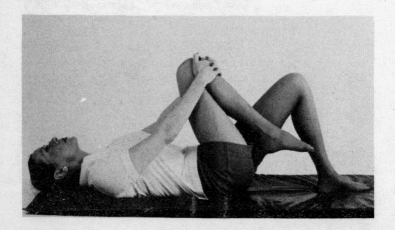

With fingers clasped around the knees, raise your head to touch the knees. Don't strain. With practice, tight muscles will stretch. Hold for five counts while breathing deeply. Repeat five times.

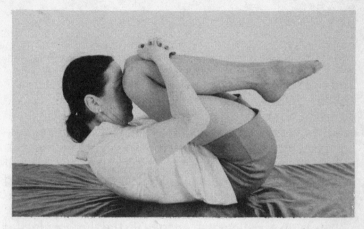

With knees bent and apart, hold the right knee with the right hand. Move it out toward the right in a large circle so the thigh will rotate in the hip socket. Repeat five times toward the right, five times toward the left. Breathe deeply during these movements. Repeat with the left leg.

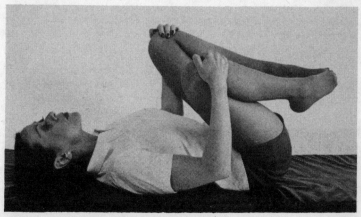

ABDOMINAL LIFT

You can do this exercise sitting or standing. Place hands on the knees, and bend slightly forward. Exhale vigorously through the mouth in a *ha* sound. This will create a vacuum in the abdominal cavity. *Without inhaling* (not easy at first) forcibly contract abdominal muscles by drawing up the diaphragm, pressing it against the rib cage so that the abdomen is pulled in and up toward the spine. Hold for ten counts *without breathing*. Repeat ten times.

This is an excellent way to tone up the three wide, flat sheets of muscles that support the abdomen; it also stimulates a sluggish colon.

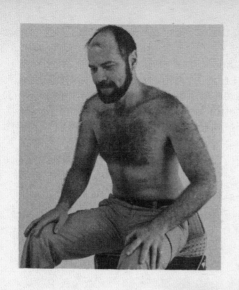

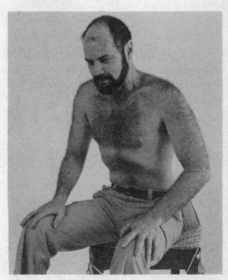

RESISTANCE EXERCISES

In this series of exercises, one muscle is pitted against the other to help tone and firm the abdomen, back, and buttocks. They are done sitting down. Repeat each one five times. For maximum benefit, hold your breath for ten counts when using resistance.

Tightening the Abdomen

Place hands just above the belt, right hand grasping the left wrist. With resistance, *pull in*, using your arm muscles. At the same time *force out* the abdominal muscles.

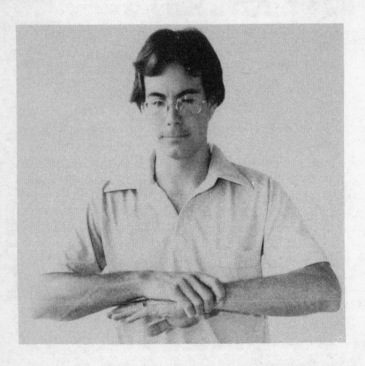

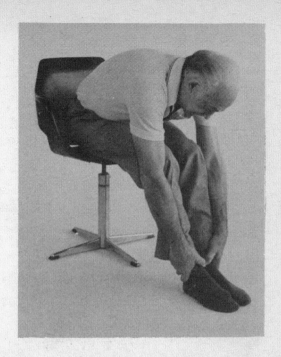

Flexing the Spine

Lean forward to grasp your legs. Bend as far as you can without straining. Flex the muscles in your back by gently stretching your arms farther down along the legs. Then slowly pull straight up, using resistance to feel the stretch along your back muscles.

Tightening the Buttocks

Sit with legs outstretched and crossed at the ankles. Hold on to the seat of the chair. Try to pull your feet apart using resistance.

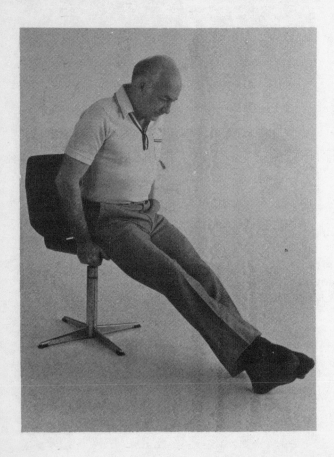

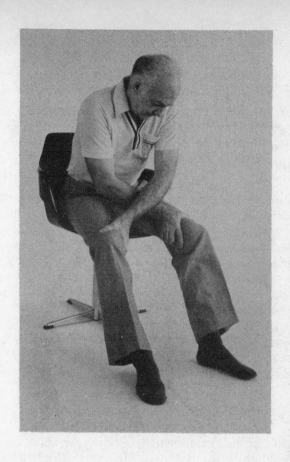

Tightening Buttocks and Inner Thighs

Lean forward slightly, with feet a few inches apart.
Cross arms and place the right hand inside the left knee,
the left hand inside the right knee. Try to press your
knees together while pushing them apart with your
hands.

HIPS, LEGS, AND FEET

LIMBERING THE KNEES

The knee is a hinge and a weight-bearing joint. Its motion is much more limited than that of most other joints. It has two cartilages, the inner and outer. When they are strong you can extend your leg fully with the knee straight. Weak cartilages cannot sustain an injury to the joint. Sudden twisting or wrenching may result in detachment of the cartilage. This kind of injury, common among football players, can be quite painful.

The knees, like the spine, show stiffness with advancing years if they are not exercised regularly. You can limber tight knees and strengthen them as well by doing the exercises on the following pages.

FENCER'S LUNGE

Stretch your left leg forward, bending the knee. Turn the toes in slightly for balance. Stretch the right leg back with knee straight, toes pointing right, and heel slightly raised. Left hand is on the left knee, right hand on the right side of the waist. Keep the back straight. Stretch as far forward as you can, bending the left knee, allowing the torso to sink down, and stretching the right leg. Then bounce up and down gently in that position to feel the stretch. Do this exercise ten times, alternating right and left legs.

Your knees, hips, and back muscles will benefit by this exercise.

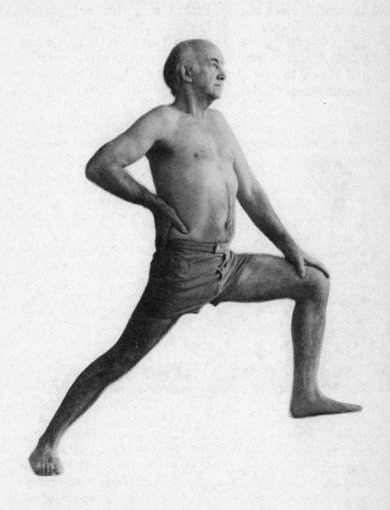

LOOSENING TIGHT KNEES

Sit on a firm, small cushion to raise the buttocks. Bend the left leg over the right thigh, or as far as it will go. *Don't force.* Hold on to the knee and ankle with both hands. Gently press down on the knee. Hold for ten counts. Relax. Stretch the left leg out, then bounce it up and down to stimulate circulation. Repeat the same movements with the right leg bent over the left thigh.

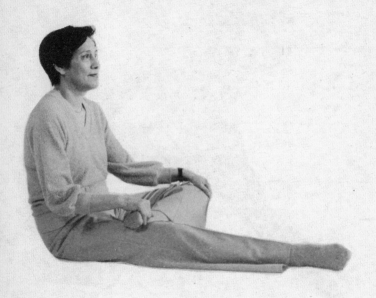

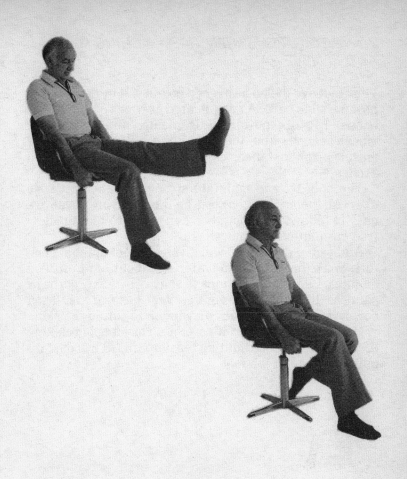

STRENGTHENING THE KNEECAP

Hold on to the sides of a chair, keeping your feet flat on the floor. Raise the left leg until the knee is straight. Contract the kneecap by pulling muscles upward, keeping the knee straight. Hold for fifteen to twenty counts. Then bend the leg down under the chair as far as possible. Hold for ten counts, and return to original position. Repeat these movements ten times, alternating right and left legs.

WAYS TO STRENGTHEN TIRED, ACHING FEET AND RELIEVE PAIN

Your feet are the basis of good posture: they deserve the best possible care. A complicated network of twenty-six bones, fifty-six powerful ligaments, and thirty-eight muscles keeps the foot in proper alignment. Weak muscles, for instance, can cause 'flat feet' or 'fallen arches.'

The only way to maintain strong, healthy feet is to exercise them. The exercises on the following pages are easy to follow, and should be done in bare feet to allow free circulation and movement.

Additional daily care will give your feet optimal comfort. Soak them in warm water for about ten to fifteen minutes. Use a pumice stone to shave down any corns or calluses by rubbing it gently over these areas. Then cover your feet with a creamy lotion to soften the skin.

Have a foot massage, if possible. This deeply relaxing therapy will release built-up tension caused by constant pain centered in the feet.

STRENGTHENING FEET AND TOES

Hold each exercise for five counts and repeat five times slowly.

Sit erect, holding on to the sides of a chair or bench. Raise heels, toes resting on the floor. Press down on the toes. The higher you raise your heels the more pull you will feel in the insteps and ankles.

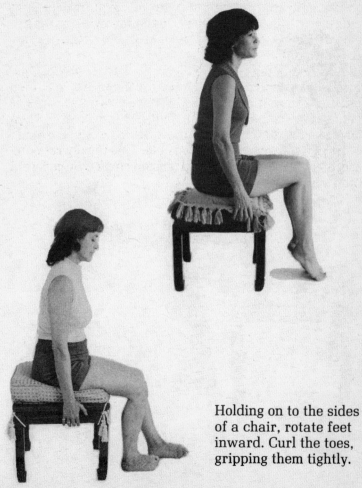

Holding on to the sides of a chair, rotate feet inward. Curl the toes, gripping them tightly.

ANKLE ROTATION

Raise left leg and rotate the ankle five times slowly toward the right, and five times toward the left without stopping. Repeat with right leg.

This exercise can also be done lying down with one leg raised and the other stretched out.

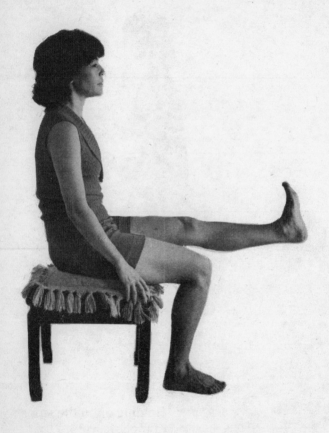

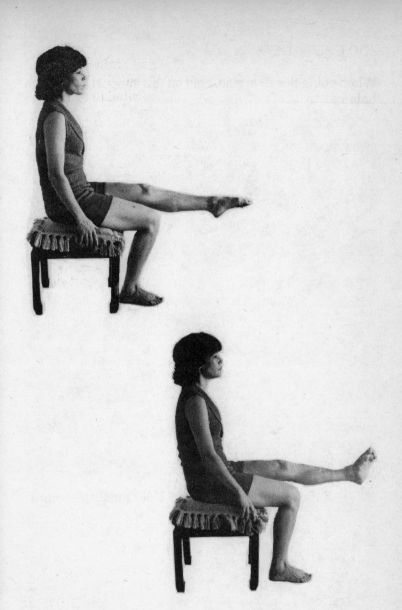

FOOT ROTATION

When doing this exercise, hold on to a support for secure balance.

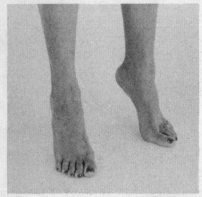

Rise up on toes.
Hold for three counts.

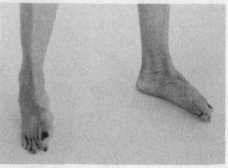

Rotate feet to outer sides. Hold for three counts.

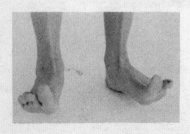

Balance on heels.
Hold for three counts.

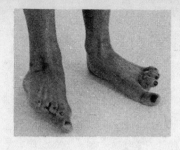

Turn feet inward.
Hold for three counts.

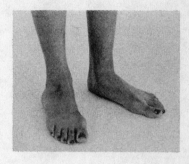

Lower feet. Hold
for three counts.

Relax for three counts and then repeat the series ten times, slowly.

HIP ROTATION

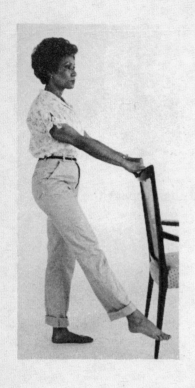 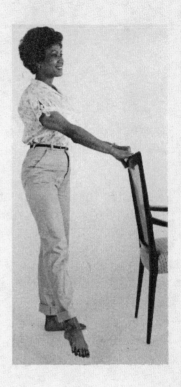

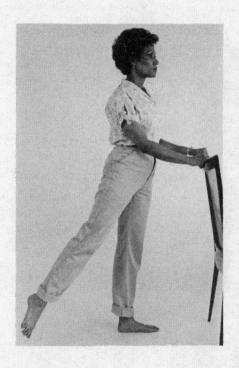

Hold on to the back of a chair. Raise right leg in front without bending the knee.

Move it slowly to the side, then back in a full circle, returning the leg to the front.

Repeat ten times slowly. Do the same movements with the left leg.

HIP STRETCH

Stand with feet apart, hands at sides. Bend to the left, sliding left hand down along the outer side of the left leg as far as possible. Straighten up. Repeat ten times. Do the same movements bending to the right. This side movement strengthens the muscles along the sides of the spine as well as stretching the hips.

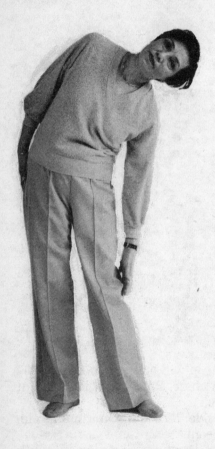

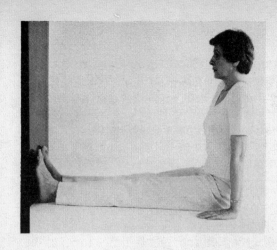

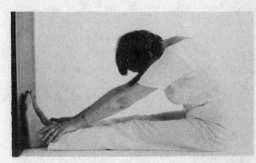

SITTING HAMSTRING STRETCH

Sit on the floor with legs outstretched and together, feet pressed against a wall. Bend forward from the hips as far as possible while stretching your arms out toward your toes. Bounce forward gently, and at the same time try to touch your toes. This will stretch the hamstring muscles in the back of your thighs. Repeat ten times.

If you have a stiff back, bounce forward gently with arms resting on your legs, just as far as you can reach. This will strengthen the upper back while stretching thigh and calf muscles. *Don't force.*

STANDING HAMSTRING STRETCH

Stand on the left leg in front of a sturdy support, such as the back of a chair, a bench, or the edge of a table. Raise the right leg and stretch it out, with heel on the support, toes pointing up. Bend forward from the hip, reaching toward your outstretched foot with both hands. Gently bounce your torso twenty times to reach farther toward your foot each time. Repeat with the left leg stretched out on the support.

If you have a stiff back, bounce your torso toward the stretched leg without straining your spine to increase the range of flexibility. Bounce twenty times toward the right leg, then repeat with the left leg.

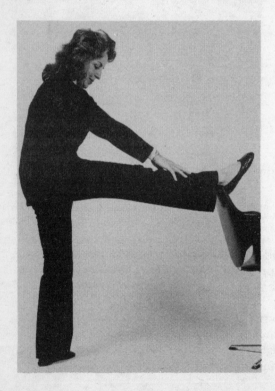

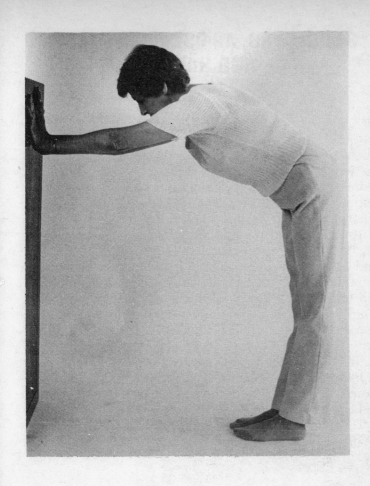

CALF-MUSCLE STRETCH

Stand facing a wall with arms stretched out, palms pressing on the wall. Keep feet together with toes pointing straight ahead, heels down. Move your pelvis (the basinlike cavity in the lower part of the trunk) forward in short jerky movements to feel a pull in the calf muscles. Repeat twenty times slowly.

SHOULDERS, ARMS, NECK, CHEST, AND HANDS

LIMBERING SHOULDER JOINTS

The shoulders have the widest range of movement of all the joints. Vigorous actions of the arm—as in bowling, tennis, or baseball—can result in damage to the tendons and tissues. Painful tendons also occur in older people whose joints are worn through aging.

Tendinitis and bursitis are common ailments which involve structures that surround the joint of the tendons and bursae. The bursa acts as a cushion for the tendon. Bursitis can occur independently of tendinitis, often in the elbow, hip, and knee (commonly known as housemaid's knee). In a bursitis attack every movement becomes extremely painful. Rest is important during this crucial period, but the affected joint should not be kept entirely immobile for too long; curtailment of the range of movement may result in a 'frozen shoulder.' Begin to exercise gradually until the shoulder joints regain their full range of motion.

The exercises given for limbering shoulder joints can be done standing or sitting.

INCREASING THE RANGE OF SHOULDER MOVEMENTS

Repeat this series five times slowly while holding each movement for five counts to feel the stretches. *Don't force.*

Place fingers on shoulders. Press arms close to the body. Relax. Lower arms.

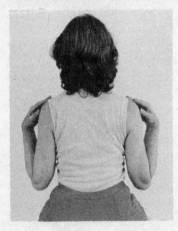

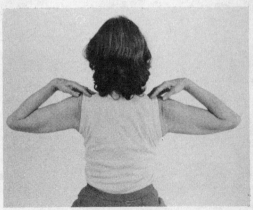

Raise arms to the sides. Tense shoulders, pulling on back muscles. Relax. Lower arms.

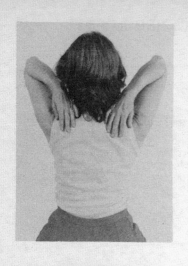
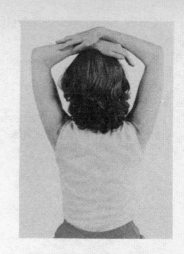

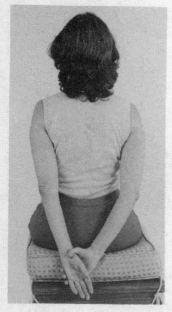
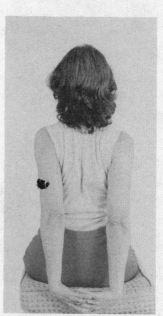

Place hands on back of shoulders, stretching arms upward. Relax. Lower arms.

Place one hand over the other, resting them on the head. Press downward, pulling on shoulder muscles. Relax. Lower arms.

With right hand clasp wrist of left hand. Pull downward while stretching shoulder and back muscles. Repeat with left hand clasping right wrist. Relax.

Interlock fingers behind back. Straighten arms away from the body while stretching shoulder and back muscles. Relax.

SHOULDER ROTATION

Repeat five times slowly while holding each movement for five counts to feel the stretches.

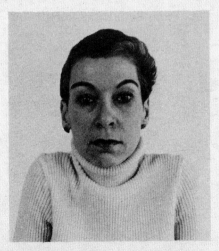

Shrug your shoulders as high as you can.

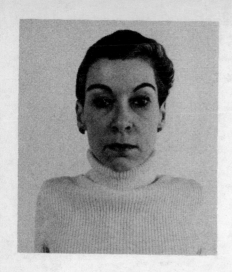

Arch them back,
pulling shoulder
blades together.

Press shoulders down.

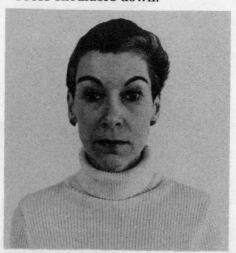

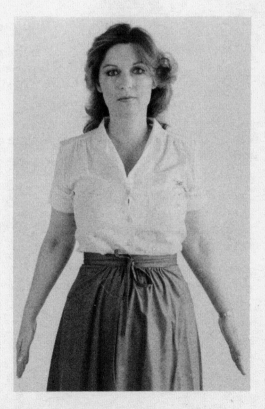

ARM STRETCHES

VERTICAL ARM STRETCH

Inhale deeply, slowly raising arms,

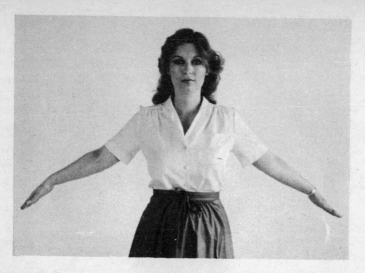

stretching them out to the sides,

then raising them higher until they are overhead. Stretch while holding the breath. Exhale and
return arms downward.

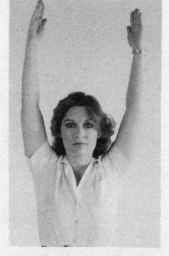

Repeat five times slowly.

HORIZONTAL ARM STRETCH

Repeat five times slowly.

Bend arms and place them close to the chest, fingertips touching.

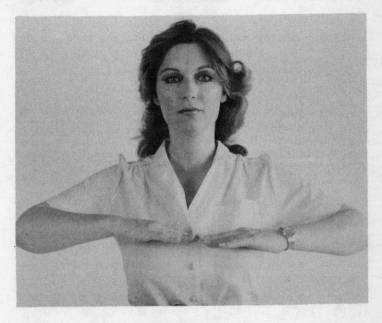

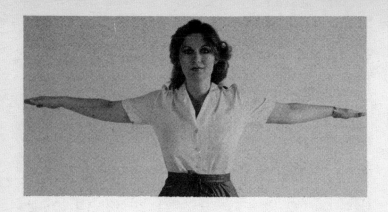

Inhale deeply while stretching arms to the sides, palms down. Hold your breath while tensing the muscles. Exhale.

Clench fists. Inhale deeply. Hold your breath while tensing the muscles. Exhale. Return to original position.

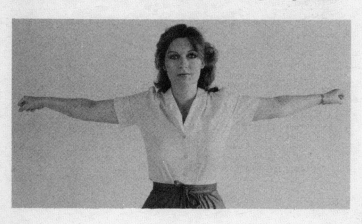

SCARF STRETCH

Repeat each stretch ten times, alternating sides. Gradually increase to twenty times.

Hold scarf ends with both hands. Stretch left arm out with right arm close to body. Pull to feel the stretch. Then stretch right arm out with left arm close to body. Pull to feel the stretch.

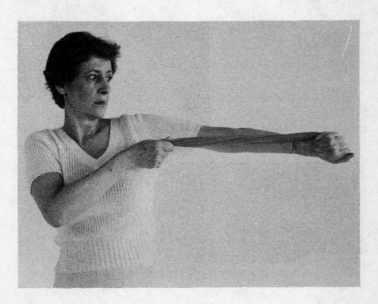

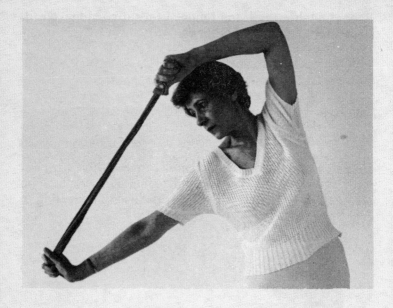

Hold scarf ends with both hands. Raise left arm over the head. Right arm is straight out. Pull downward to feel the stretch. Then raise left arm over the head. Right arm is straight out. Pull downward to feel the stretch.

BACK SCARF STRETCH

This is an effective way to increase range of movement in the shoulders and limber the arms, while at the same time improving the posture.

Hold scarf ends with both hands behind the back, right hand up, left hand down. To increase your stretch, grip tightly onto both ends of the scarf as you inch your fingers toward the center. With repeated practice you might eventually be able to interlock your fingers or reach much closer. Repeat this exercise ten times. Then reverse movements with left hand up, right hand down.

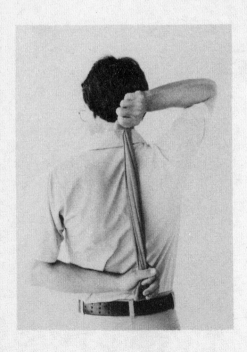

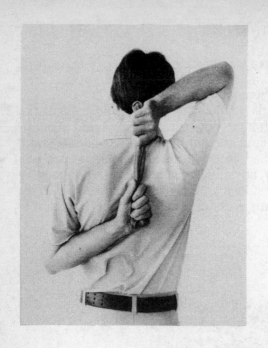

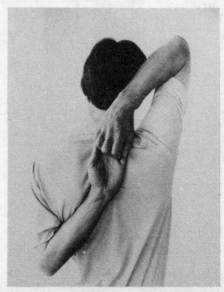

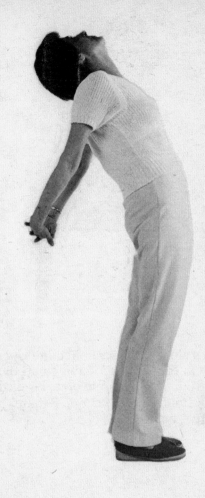

BACK STRETCH

Stand with legs slightly apart. Interlock fingers behind
your back. Inhale and at the same time stretch arms
back and out. To feel the stretch, arch the neck back.
Hold for five counts. Exhale and relax. Repeat five times.

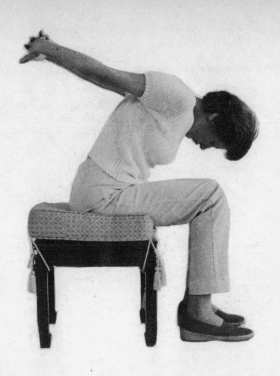

Sit on a stool with legs apart. Interlock fingers behind your back. Inhale and at the same time stretch arms back and out. To feel the stretch, lower the head as arms come up. Hold for five counts. Exhale. Sit up and relax. Repeat five times.

LOOSENING TIGHT NECK MUSCLES

NECK STRETCH

Drop your head limply forward to stretch the back of the
neck. Hold for five counts, then lift your head slowly and
drop it back to stretch your throat. Hold again for five
counts. Repeat six times.

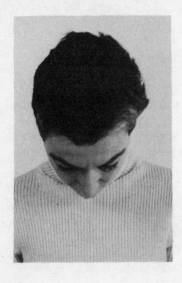

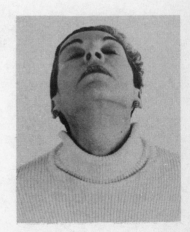

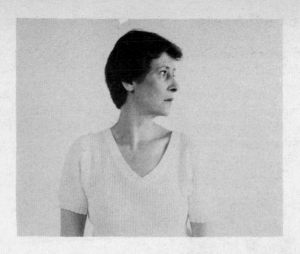

Turn your head to the extreme right, looking over the shoulder (without moving the shoulders). Hold for five counts. Then turn your head to the extreme left, looking over the shoulder. Hold for five counts. Repeat six times.

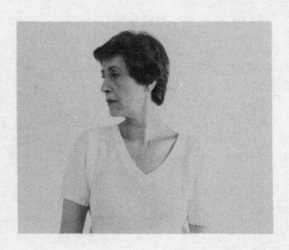

NECK ROTATION

Roll your head slowly and loosely in a wide circle: forward and down, right, back, left, forward. Repeat five times.

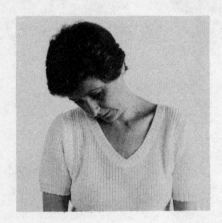

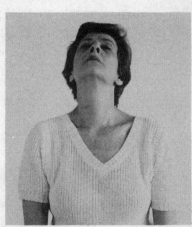

Reverse the motion. Breathe freely. Take a deep breath after you have completed the fifth rolling motion.

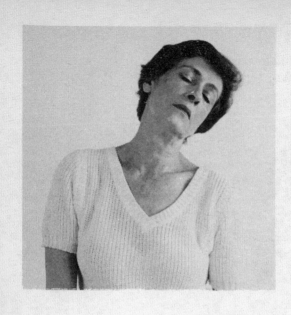

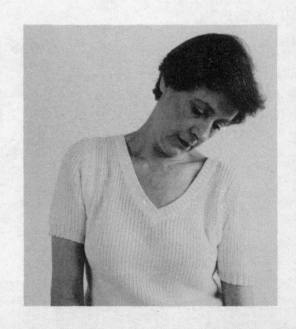

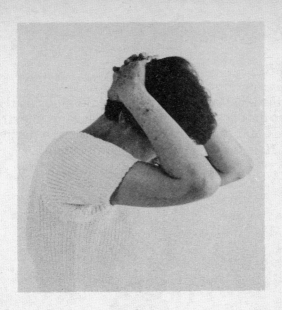

NECK PULL

Clasp hands behind the head, fingers interlocked. With resistance, pitting one muscle against the other, bring the head forward. You should feel the pull in the neck and shoulders. Hold for five counts. Repeat ten times.

TONING THE PECTORAL MUSCLES

FIST PRESS

Bend the elbows and place the right fist inside the left, close to the chest. Press together, using forcible strength of arms and shoulders, pitting one muscle against the other. Hold for ten counts. Repeat five times.

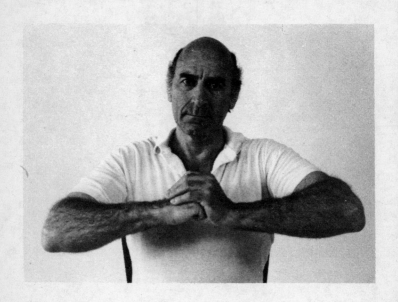

ELBOW PRESS

Clasp hands behind the head, fingers interlocked. Stretch elbows as far back as possible, bringing the shoulder blades together. Hold for five counts to feel the pull in the chest, ribs, shoulder blades, and spine. Repeat five times.

This is also a chest stretch to improve posture and tone the pectoral (chest) muscles.

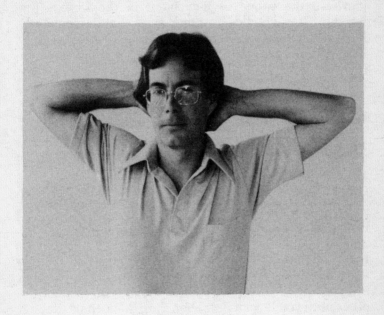

FOR FINGERS AND WRISTS

The twenty-seven bones in each hand and wrist represent a fourth of the bones in the entire body. Thousands of nerve endings are heavily concentrated in the fingertips, causing them to become extremely sensitive when injured. When the joints are stiff and swollen and our hands don't function as they normally should, we feel paralyzed. The exercises on pages 126 to 134 will help to increase the range of movement in the fingers and wrists. They should be done slowly and frequently. Repeat the exercises with both hands; first separately, then together.

HAND STRETCH

Hold each movement for five counts.

Forcefully spread the fingers apart. Hold while stretching each finger to its full length and span. Draw them inward with resistance, pitting one muscle against the other until you form a fist. Then fling them apart. Repeat five times.

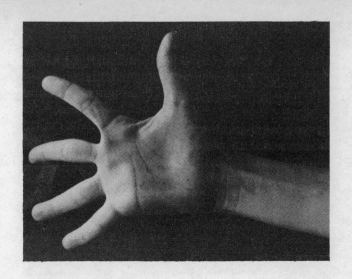

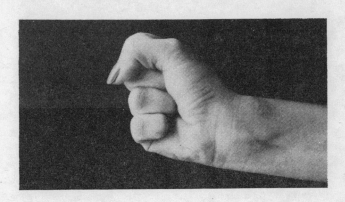

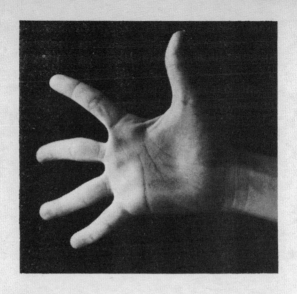

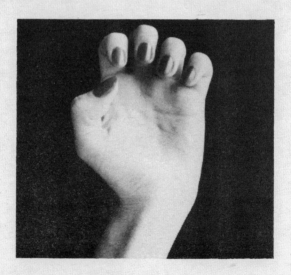

Spread the fingers apart, then bend them at the joints, pressing firmly. Repeat five times.

FINGER FLEXIBILITY # 1

Hold each movement for five counts.
 Spread the fingers apart. Stretch each one to its full length.

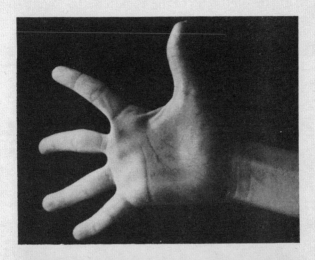

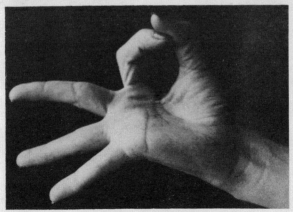

Touch the tip of the thumb to the top of the nail of the index finger. Press firmly. Keep other fingers stretched apart.

With the index finger turned in toward the palm, touch the tip of the thumb to the middle finger. Press firmly. Keep other fingers stretched apart.

With the index and middle fingers turned in toward the palm, touch the tip of the thumb to the fourth finger. Keep little finger stretched out.

Then turn the little finger in toward the palm. Press firmly with the thumb. Clench the fist tightly. Fling the fingers apart.

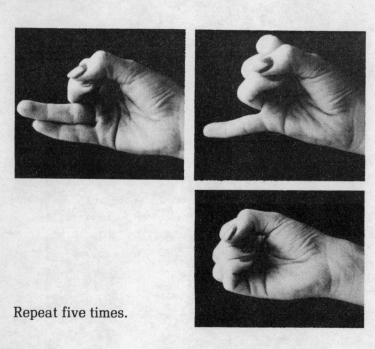

Repeat five times.

FINGER FLEXIBILITY # 2

Hold each movement for five counts.

Fingers are together, outstretched, thumb pointing up. Turn the fifth finger inward toward the palm. Keep the other fingers as straight as possible. Then turn in the fourth, third, and index fingers, stretching each one slowly. Close the thumb over the fingers, pressing tightly. Reverse the movements: stretch the thumb out, followed by the fingers.

Repeat five times.

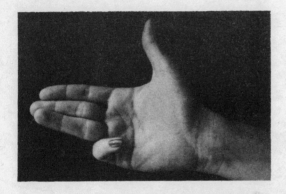

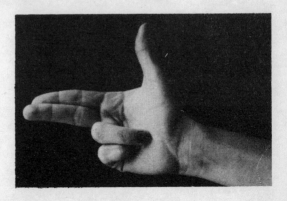

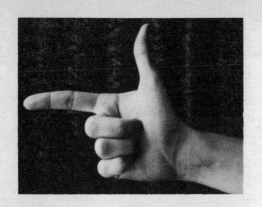

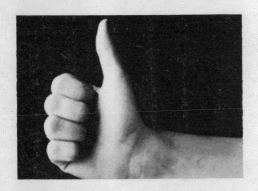

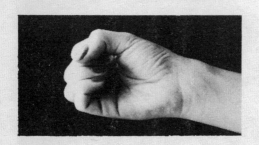

FINGER STRETCH

Hold each movement for five counts.

Grasp the right index finger with left hand. Press back and down gently. Repeat five times with each finger, including the thumb. Do the same movements with the left hand.

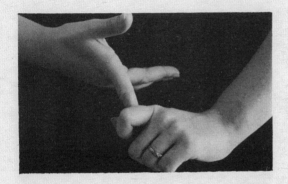

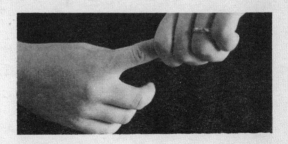

Grasp the right index finger with left hand. Gently rotate the finger five times slowly toward the right, five times toward the left. Repeat the movements with each finger, adding a little more pressure to increase the range of motion. Do the same movements with the left hand.

WRIST ROTATION

Grasp right hand just above the wrist with left hand. Gently rotate the right wrist five times slowly toward the right, five times toward the left. Repeat the movements, adding a little more pressure to increase the range of motion. Reverse hands and rotate left wrist. If your wrists are painful, do this exercise very gently.

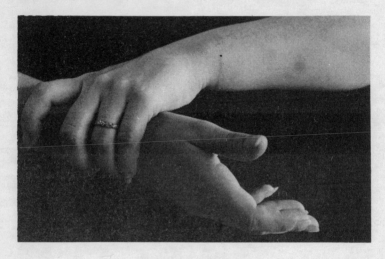

PASSIVE EXERCISES

Anyone can help you with these passive exercises, which will bring relief to painful joints and increase the range of motion. The instructions are addressed to the helper. The movements must be done slowly, using gentle pressure to manipulate the joints.

FINGER MANIPULATIONS (also excellent for toes)

Repeat five times slowly.

Grasp wrist with one hand. With the other, press the thumb slightly back, then forward. Repeat with each finger.

Rotate the thumb and index fingers separately in a circular motion.

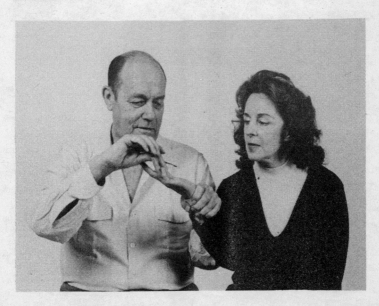

FOR THE ARMS AND SHOULDERS

Repeat each exercise five times slowly. Hold each movement for five counts.

Raise arm to the side. Hold, then lower it.

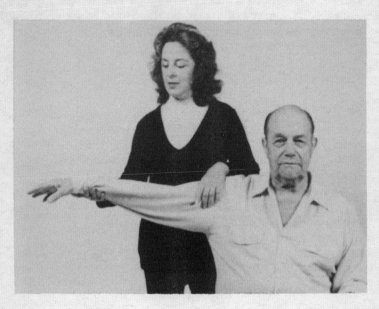

Bend the elbow using gentle pressure until hand is above the shoulder, or as far as it will go. Hold. Stretch arm out, then lower it.

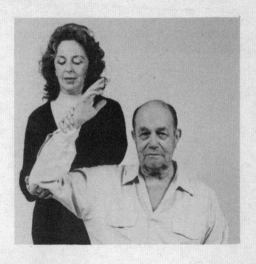

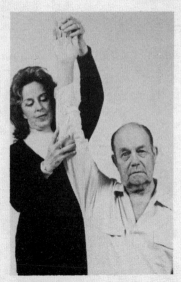

Raise arm upward, pulling gently. Hold, then lower it.

Raise both arms as high as possible.
Hold, then lower them.

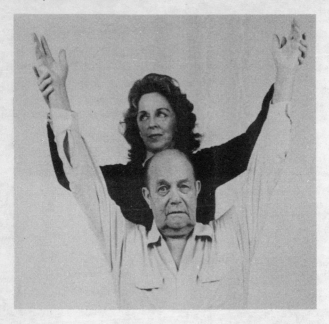

Bend elbows so palms of hands touch the chest. Hold, then lower them.

Bend elbows so hands are above the shoulders. Hold, then lower them.

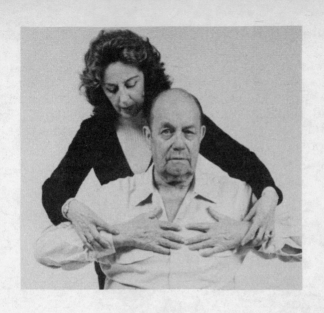

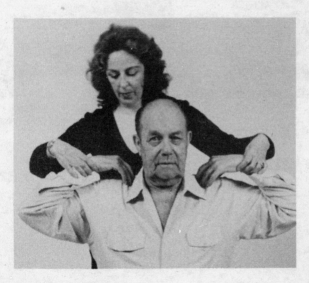

FOR THE LEGS AND HIPS

On the back:

Raise one leg as high as possible with the other on the mat. Hold for five counts. Then rotate the leg in a wide circle to loosen the hip socket. Repeat ten times slowly. Lower leg to the mat. Repeat with other leg.

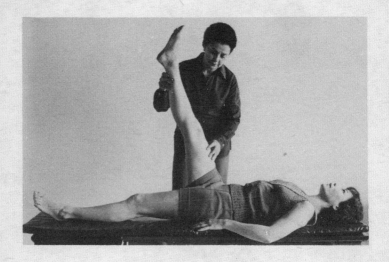

Grasp both legs and raise them off the mat. Bend the knees, then straighten them. Repeat twenty times slowly without stopping. Lower legs to the mat.

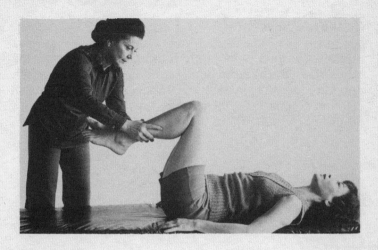

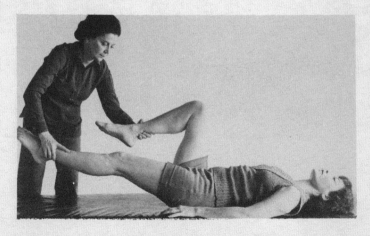

Grasp both legs and raise them off the mat. Bend one knee and straighten it, then bend the other knee and straighten it. Repeat this motion slowly without stopping for twenty counts. Lower legs to mat.

On the abdomen:

Subject lies face down, one hand under the head, the other down at the side. Bend leg as far back as possible, applying gentle pressure. Other leg should remain relaxed. Repeat ten times slowly. Lower leg. Repeat with other leg.

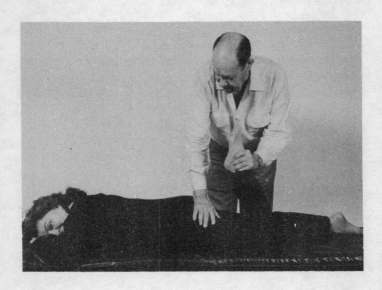

Do the same exercise bending both legs together.

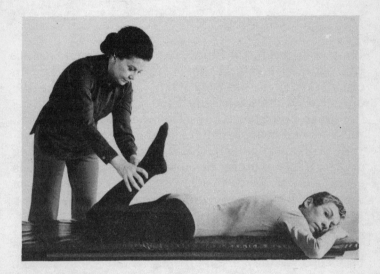

7 THE JOY OF WALKING

Walking is a natural fitness exercise that most people can enjoy. It keeps all the muscles in tone, steps up circulation, gives the body fluidity of motion, helps the digestive system, lowers the blood pressure, strengthens the lungs and heart, and releases tension. It is both relaxing and invigorating for the mind and body.

By walking regularly, you can slow down the aging process. This exercise firms sagging bodies and burns extra calories. Lean muscle tissue replaces fat. If you are among the millions of people who sit or stand for long periods, walking will ease the aches and pains of your joints and muscles.

You will need a pair of good shoes. Running shoes are best because they are light-weight and roomy for the toes, with well-cushioned heels, good heel grip, and arch supports. Wear thick socks to absorb perspiration and reduce friction.

It is easier to walk in loose, comfortable clothes than in tight-fitting garments that restrict movement. In winter, a light waterproof jacket over a sweater will protect your chest and back, and a woolen cap or hat will absorb perspiration from your head, keeping it warm.

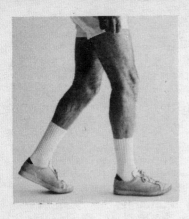 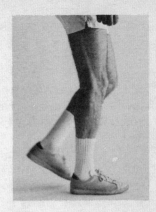

In walking correctly, the heel strikes down first, then the weight shifts to the ball of the foot and rolls onto the toes.

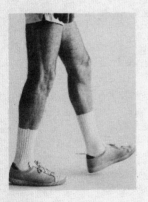 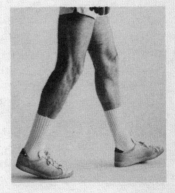

Walking should be pleasurable, never tiring to the point of exhaustion. Walk as briskly as you can. Develop a rhythm. Let your arms swing freely down, toes pointing straight ahead. The forward swing of your legs, which involves the hip, knee, and heel, ends with the heel striking down first. The weight then shifts to the ball of the foot and rolls onto the toes. Practice the foot movements slowly to get the right rhythm: the heel strikes down first, then the weight shifts to the ball of the foot and rolls onto the toes.

The exercises given in Chapter 6, 'Hips, Legs, and Feet,' are most helpful for building up your stamina. It is best to do some conditioning exercises before you set out on your walk to avoid the tightening up of muscles, tendons, and ligaments along the backs of the legs.

Long walks may be too stressful for joints of the knees or ankles if they are swollen. Consult your doctor about it.

Take it easy at first if you are not accustomed to physical exercise. Build up your stamina slowly, and increase your distance gradually. Start out walking for about ten to fifteen minutes. Make it more enjoyable by picking routes that are free of heavy traffic and noise.

Some people walk with natural grace, others have a labored style. Even if you must walk with a cane, you can get the most out of this exercise by breathing rhythmically and coordinating the breathing with the movements of your arms and legs. This will give you a lighter, springier step. As you inhale through your nostrils, take three or four normal strides, then as you exhale through your mouth (for a quicker supply of oxygen) take the same number of steps. When you get into the spirit of walking you will develop your own pace and rhythm, and you will enjoy the fresh air your lungs take in. Your muscles will feel stretched and relaxed as the blood circulates more freely.

EPILOGUE

This book carries a strong message: you can bring about significant changes in your life simply by taking the first step to help yourself. It is hard to be rational when you are suffering, but the more you concentrate on pain the more you will feel it, since pain is perceived in the brain. People who are seriously ill are naturally depressed, but it is the perception of these misfortunes that determines the degree of the illness. It is a known fact that negative emotions of fear, hate, anger, or anxiety can weaken the body's defenses against disease. Positive emotions have the reverse effect.

In his book, *Free Yourself of Pain*, David E. Bresden, Ph.D., former director of the pain control unit of the University of California Medical Center, has said that people with chronic pain often don't do things they would normally enjoy. They feel they can't because of the pain, but it is often the other way around. Their pain persists because they aren't having any fun.

You have within you the resources to rise above the pain and depression that are holding you prisoner. Think about it this way: when you are obsessed with negative emotions, you are much like the weary traveler burdened by excess baggage. Throw off this weight and be free. There are bound to be days when you are cast down in despair. At these times take your mind off yourself and concentrate on some pleasurable pursuit—a funny film, a good book, work you enjoy—or be among people who can bring laughter into your life. Norman Cousins, author of *Anatomy of an Illness*, found that laughter had a salutary effect on the apparently incurable disease that he eventually conquered. Humor is one of the oldest and simplest of therapies. When you can

147

laugh and are happy you feel optimistic and positive. A positive attitude toward yourself brings about positive actions, increasing your energy level and your determination to overcome adversity.

You will need the courage to begin. Ignore the mental signals that say, 'I can't.' You will need the courage to persist when progress seems slow or nonexistent. Your mind will continually provide you with reasons to give up. It will tell you: 'It's not doing me any good . . . I think I may be making things worse . . . I'm more stiff today than I was yesterday . . . I haven't the time . . . It's boring.' Be prepared for the explosion of excuses to which your mind will subject you. They are false messages.

Don't try to tackle too much at the start. Set a modest goal. It's your body. You are the only one who can select the exercises that will be the most helpful. Experiment. If one part of your body is particularly stiff and painful—a shoulder, a hip, a knee—work on that gently. When it feels better, you will realize that you have the power to help yourself. Little by little, day by day, you will see some improvements in your body and in your state of mind. Changes that seem miraculous can be made to happen if you have the will to achieve them.

INDEX

mental energy, improvement of
    through deep breathing, 40
Menuhin, Yehudi, 18
Michelangelo, 34
mind-control, 20–21, 55–60
    concentration improved by, 24
    exercises for, 56–60
    meditation and, 21, 24, 56
    mood drugs vs., 55
    sitting positions in, 56
    yoga and, 20, 55
muscle relaxants, 18
muscles:
    anterior view of, 36
    heart as, 38
    posterior view of, 37
    skeletal (voluntary), 38
    smooth (involuntary), 38
    weakened, 34

neck, exercises for, 119–23
Neck Pull, 123
Neck Rotation, 121–2
Neck Stretch, 119–20
nerves, pressure on, 17, 63
nervous system, autonomic, 38
Newton, Isaac, 30
Numeral Concentration, 58–9
nutrition, 30–32
    alcohol and, 30, 31
    basic foods in, 30–31
    coffee and, 31
    dieting and, 31–2
    emotional factors in, 31
    raw and whole foods in, 31
    tea and, 31
    vitamins and, 30
    water and, 31

organs affected by arthritis,
    29
osteoarthritis, 17, 26–7, 28
    Herberden's Nodes in, 27, 28
    heredity and, 27
    injuries and, 17, 27
    osteophytes in, 27

in postmenopausal females,
    27
    primary, 27
    secondary, 27
    treatment of, 27
osteophytes, 27
Overall Flexibility, 79–81
overexercise, hazards of, 33
oxygen:
    of brain, 40
    deep breathing and, 40, 41–2

pain:
    depression and, 17, 27, 29,
        147, 148
    laughter and, 147–8
    positive emotions and, 147–8
    as warning, 32, 33, 62
passive exercises, 135–43
    for arms, 136–9
    for fingers, 135
    gentle pressure in, 135
    for hips, 140–43
    for legs, 140–43
    for shoulders, 136–9
    for toes, 135
    see also exercise
pectoral muscles, exercises for,
    124
Pelvic Stretch, 72–3
posture:
    in sitting, 63, 66–7
    in standing, 65–6
prana, 55

Resistance Breathing, 48–50
Resistance Exercises, 84–7
respiratory ailments, 41
rest, 33
rheumatoid arthritis, 17, 26,
    27–9
    genetic markers of, 27
    symptoms of, 27
    treatment of, 27, 29
Rib-Cage Breathing, 42, 45
Rodin, Auguste, 34

THE POCKET HOLIDAY DOCTOR
by Caroline Chapman & Caroline Lucas BM BCh

All the dos and don'ts for a healthy holiday . . .

How to keep the family free from holiday hazards . . .

How to cope with sickness, diarrhoea, sunburn, bites, fever, etc, etc

Zero hour . . . when to recognise you must have a doctor . . . and how to find one in any language . . .

How this book came to be written . . .

One of the authors, Caroline Chapman, found herself in a mother's nightmare. In an idyllic holiday home, her ten year old child developed a temperature of 103° and had diarrhoea so severe she was passing blood. They had no transport. The nearest telephone was half a mile away, the nearest doctor ten miles and he couldn't speak English.

There and then Caroline Chapman vowed that if her daughter pulled through she would write a book offering practical advice . . .

Here, from Caroline Chapman and Dr Caroline Lucas, is a book for emergencies of all kinds, from the simple sting of a jelly fish, to a possible outbreak of cholera . . .

0 552 121959   £1.25

SEXUAL HEALTH AND FITNESS FOR WOMEN
by Kathryn Lance and Maria Agardy

A NEW WAY TO SEXUAL AND REPRODUCTIVE WELL-BEING

Sexual Health and Fitness for Women tells you how to:

*Be more responsive sexually

*Have more and better orgasms

*Relieve menstrual pain and pre-menstrual tension

*Achieve easier childbirth and recovery and at the same time how to:

*Flatten your stomach

*Streamline your bottom

*Firm your inner thighs

*Build muscles that fight backache

and much more . . . This is the first book, written by women for women, to tell you everything you need to know about strengthening your pelvic girdle. General exercise won't do it. But this proven three-phase programme will!

0 552 990116   £1.95

THE BEVERLY HILLS EXERCISE BOOK
by Roberta Krech with Bill Libby

YOU CAN LEARN THE SECRETS OF BEAUTY AND FITNESS THAT, UNTIL NOW, ONLY THE ELITE COULD AFFORD

From her exclusive Beverly Hills salon, physical-fitness and skin-care expert Roberta Krech invites you to experience the simple, natural exercise programme that gives her rich and famous clients their youthful looks and slim, supple figures.

Ms Krech will show you how to "steal" a few minutes here and there throughout your day for the quick and easy excercises that will keep you trim, toned and energized. Wherever you are, from morning till midnight, her fabulous star-proven system will shape-up your entire body — face and neck, shoulders and upper arms, bust and back, waist and abdomen, hips and buttocks, thighs and calves, ankles and feet . . . and there's never a boring caisthenic to do!

With personal beauty tips and professional skin care instructions, plus exercises to share and relaxation techniques, THE BEVERLY HILLS EXERCISE BOOK allows you to attain the radiant and glowing beauty of the fashionable women of Beverly Hills.

12158 4   £1.75

A SELECTION OF DIET, HEALTH AND EXERCISE BOOKS AVAILABLE FROM CORGI

While every effort is made to keep prices low, it is sometimes necessary to increase prices at short notice. Corgi Books reserve the right to show new retail prices on covers which may differ from those previously advertised in the text or elsewhere.

The prices shown below were correct at the time of going to press.

☐ 12158 4	**The Beverly Hills Exercise Book**	*Roberta Krech*	£1.75
☐ 23148 0	**Getting Well Again**	*Carl & Stephanie Simonton*	£1.95
☐ 01435 8	**Jane Brody's Nutrition Book**	*Jane Brody*	£4.95
☐ 10336 5	**The Magic of Honey**	*Barbara Cartland*	£1.50
☐ 12195 9	**The Pocket Holiday Doctor**	*Caroline Chapman &*	
		Dr. Caroline Lucas	£1.25
☐ 11637 8	**Common Childhood Illnesses**	*Dr. David Delvin*	£1.25
☐ 14437 5	**Nutrition and Vitamin Therapy**	*Dr. Michael Lesser M.D.*	£1.25
☐ 01409 9	**Infant Massage**	*Vimala Schneider*	£1.95
☐ 12155 X	**The G Spot**	*Alice Kahn Ladas,*	
		Beverly Whipple & John Perry	£1.95
☐ 99011 6	**Sexual Health and Fitness for Women**	*Kathryn Lance &*	
		Maria Agardy	£1.95

ORDER FORM

All these books are available at your book shop or newsagent or can be ordered direct from the publisher. Just tick the titles you want and fill in the form below.

CORGI BOOKS, Cash Sales Department, P.O. Box 11, Falmouth, Cornwall.

Please send cheque or postal order, no currency.

Please allow cost of book(s) plus the following for postage and packing:

U.K. Customers—Allow 45p for the first book, 20p for the second book and 14p for each additional book ordered, to a maximum charge of £1.63.

B.F.P.O. and Eire—Allow 45p for the first book, 20p for the second book plus 14p per copy for the next 7 books, there after 8p per book.

Overseas Customers—Allow 75p for the first book and 21p per copy for each additional book.

NAME (Block Letters) ....

ADDRESS ....

....